GRA

HO

FOR BODY, MIND & SPIRIT

GRAIL SPRINGS
HOLISTIC DETOX

FOR BODY, MIND & SPIRIT

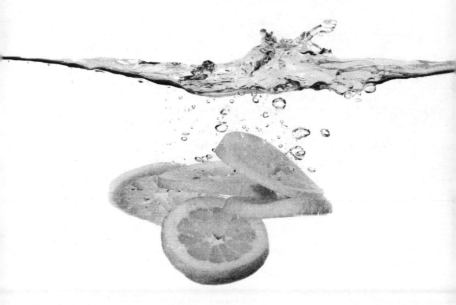

Madeleine Marentette

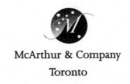

McArthur & Company

Toronto

First published in 2007 by
McArthur & Company

This paperback edition published in 2009 by
McArthur & Company
322 King St. West, Suite 402
Toronto, ON
M5V 1J2
www.mcarthur-co.com

Library and Archives Canada Cataloguing in Publication

Marentette, Madeleine
Grail Springs holistic detox : for body, mind & spirit / Madeleine Marentette ;
foreword by Elson Haas.

Includes index.
ISBN 978-1-55278-779-3

1. Grail Springs Health and Wellness Centre. 2. Detoxification (Health).
3. Self-care, Health. 4. Cookery. 5. Holistic medicine. I. Title.

RA810.B35M37 2009   613   C2009-902016-5

Design and composition by Tania Craan

Printed in Canada by Webcom

The publisher would like to acknowledge the financial support of the Government
of Canada through the Book Publishing Industry Development Program (BPIDP)
and the Canada Council for our publishing activities. The publisher further
wishes to acknowledge the financial support of the Ontario Arts Council
for our publishing program.

10 9 8 7 6 5 4 3 2 1

This book is dedicated to…

Mother Earth
For she will be well when we all are well.

and Chandra
You were perfect as you were. I miss you.

Table of Contents

Foreword

by Elson M. Haas, MD, *The Detox Doc*™

I have been to Grail Springs Wellness Centre and met with Madeleine Marentette, and am so impressed with the facility and programs that I am delighted to be able to contribute to this book and act as a consultant for the Grail. What Madeleine and her team offer people is a chance to re-create themselves and learn what it takes to live in a way that generates health, rather than the way most people live in this polluted, over-processed, and high-stress world that causes much of the disease that the typical Westerner experiences and that is so costly to our health-care systems.

When illness happens, it exists at all levels of our being — nutritional and biochemical, physical, emotional, mental (mind/body), and spiritual. Thus, when we are seeking true healing, it helps to look at and care for as many of these areas as possible. Illness represents conflict, and healing often means learning, change, and evolution. I wrote about this in the conclusion of my first book, *Staying Healthy with the Seasons*. Does our illness result from past actions and lifestyle and not living in alignment with our truth, our true selves? I think so.

From my 35 years of patient care, focusing on lifestyle correction, natural therapies in a family practice, as well as individual and group detoxification programs, I see that healing occurs and moves when we address our lives and make changes. A primary philosophy I live and practice by is this, "How we feel and look is a result of how we live; thus, if we want to look and feel better, something needs to change." When we just get treatment to control our physical symptoms with drugs as we often do in Western Medicine, we are often looking for the immediate problems/symptoms to go away; however, the underlying cause(s) are most often still present. These causes typically have to do with lifestyle – what we choose to eat, how we think and the stresses we have, our quality of sleep, how we exercise and move our body, and our attitudes toward our self and our life – which is a key. I encourage my patients and all of you to develop the following attitude, which involves a deep spiritual principle: "Treat your body with LOVE; it's the only one you have." When you do this, you are likely to eat what truly nourishes your body and provides your cells with the many nutrients they need to function optimally. You will also exercise appropriately for you to stay fit, make sure you get proper sleep, and learn ways to handle your stresses and emotions.

This process of healing often begins with detoxification – eliminating or minimizing the intake of toxins from food, air, and water while you nourish your body with wholesome fresh foods and juices. You might also begin by avoiding and taking a break from your SNACC habits – Sugar, Nicotine, Alcohol, Caffeine, and Chemicals – that surely undermine your health from your consistent and persistent use of them. Habitual use of these substances as well as refined flour products and excessive animal proteins and dairy products can cause a condition that is too acid in the body.

This leads to mucous congestion, inflammation, and eventually degenerative changes in the body, the basis of most chronic disease. We can correct this acidic condition and thus prevent and slow much disease and aging. This alkalizing/detoxification process becomes the first steps for most people, and there are many steps and layers for true healing. Yet, this becomes easiest if you think of one step at a time, and then you can really do it and not feel overwhelmed. Even with a few steps, you will begin to see and feel this improved health and vitality. And that's what a trip to the wonderful Grail Springs Wellness Centre and your journey through this book can provide.

With a focus on the purification process and the concepts of acid/alkaline body and diets, you can learn tools that can help you for life. Much of disease comes from one primary problem – cellular dysfunction. There are two causes. First is deficiency of vital nutrients – vitamins, minerals, amino acids, fatty acids, and phytonutrients from fresh foods – all of which your body and cells need to function optimally. The other cause is toxicity from exposure to not only environmental chemicals and metals like lead and mercury, but also the toxicity generated from the food choices we make, specifically overly acid foods like refined and processed flour and sugar products as well as excessive animal meats and dairy products. This acidity leads to toxicity and inflammation and eventually to degeneration and breakdown of the body's function and thus energy and vitality. These concepts and solutions are addressed fully in my popular book, *The New Detox Diet*.

For those of you who cannot make it to The Grail Springs Wellness Centre, a beautiful spot north of Toronto, this book can be a guide, a vacation, for you to embrace and utilize. Herein lies your pathway to better health

Stay Healthy,

Elson M. Haas, MD, The Detox Doc™
Integrated Medicine Practitioner
Author of many books on health and nutrition
(see www.elsonhaas.com)
Staying Healthy with the Seasons, *The New Detox Diet*,
and *Staying Healthy with Nutrition*

Introduction

The Quest for Wholeness

Imagine a life complete and utterly perfect. It is an age-old quest and, some might say, not possible. What is a complete life; what is a perfect life? Is it all subjective and relative to the perception of the viewer? Is there a universal truth and reality to this query, or is it unanswerable? It is easy to guess there would be a thousand different views from a thousand different individuals if asked. Perhaps it is found in our courage, the day we overcome a fear. Perhaps it is found in the act of discovering and moving on our passion while we say good-bye to complacency, forever. Or maybe when justice prevails over injustice, or when free expression breaks free from suppression. Is it the spinning of calm out of chaos or witnessing healthy cells replace sick cells? Could the perfection of life be the gained awareness over ignorance? Or is it simply the true joy we might come to know when we discover that every single day of our life we have the given opportunity to become restored and whole?

Perhaps it appears in both the subtle and the unassuming, from the smallest to the most profound realization. Maybe it appears as the continuous eternal stream of opportunity to overcome some one thing every moment of our life. Pure joy can be had when we embrace the act of change itself, when the virtual motion of transformation is felt within, when we see the positive results of change with our own eyes. We are complete when our body, mind, and heart are healed, conscious, connected, and whole again. Perhaps then, it is the discovery of the potential within us that is so perfect. This age-old query is the story of the legendary quest for the Holy Grail, and in my mind, it is the greatest story ever told.

> The quest is for wholeness, and the
> experience of it takes place where matter
> and spirit meet.

An Ancient Holistic Blueprint

The legendary quest for the Holy Grail is a story that was born out of a brutal time in human history, the Crusades, approximately A.D. 1000. It is a story that crosses time, peoples, religions, empires, and the imagination of just about every single person who has ever walked the planet. It is about the human journey in self-discovery and restoration. If one succeeds in this quest there is a reward. A great reward. You get to know who you really are. In a sense, you get to make the ultimate high-speed, wireless connection with God, divinity or universal intelligence!

This journey in self-realization and transformation begins as soon as we set foot on a human path which can, without a doubt, prove to be both beautiful and quite harsh and unforgiving at times. There are tests of humility, sickness, loyalty, honesty, conviction, greed, renunciation, gluttony, courage, compassion, and fortitude, to name a few. We live through these tests every single day of our life whether we choose to or not, whether we like it or not. We are faced with choices and decisions. We act. And then we get to live with the outcome. Sometimes our choices and decisions come back to bite us. Sometimes they fizzle because they lack fervour and passion. Sometimes the results are exactly what we envision, and sometimes they are beyond our wildest expectation. These tests can get harder before they get easier. It can feel as though we are walking on the razor's edge. Sometimes we want it (life) to be over. But when we persist and persevere, the rewards can outweigh the seeming price we paid.

The grail quest is woven throughout this book, as it relates to modern day life, challenges and issues, not unlike the challenges laid before Perceval and the Knights of the Round Table. The story is about each soul born into this world. It is a story about each of us. It recognizes how we are born into this world innocent, pure, and whole. Very early in our life we get knocked around, battered, and bruised, becoming messed up in the middle somewhere – emotionally, mentally, and physically. As a result, we often unconsciously and consciously hurt others, causing chaos and wreaking havoc, and live from one crisis to another. If we are lucky, towards the latter part of our life, we finally awaken to ourselves, and race to the finish line to fix that which we broke in the earlier part of our life. It is when we begin fixing everything we have broken, that we become in ourselves restored.

Be Open

Let me ask you as you read Grail Springs Holistic Detox , that you be open to contemplation and self-reflection. Let down your guard. Be free to get real with your Self. Open up your senses. See, feel, hear, and utilize your intuition and imagination. Your ability to imagine, and imagine with clarity is key. This book is not a quick fix instruction book. Our intent at Grail Springs and in this book is that you begin to open up your own intuitive sensitivities and become connected to the grander scheme of who you are and how we all fit into this life. Get connected with your body, mind, heart, spirit, and with this planet. Where we are disconnected, imbalance exists, trouble brews and the toil begins. When you are connected, there is little room for error and you are in the flow of life. And healing begins. When you are connected, you are awake to life, and brilliance lies ahead.

This is a guide for all people at all levels – whether you are just starting out or whether you are further along on the path to self knowledge and wholeness. And it matters not where you live in this world. You are the knight in this story. It is your journey as it is mine, as we quest for wholeness in our life. The reward of wholeness is yours to pursue.

Woven through these pages will be tenets of an ancient blueprint to transformation – of body, heart, and mind – for the three are interrelated. As you become more connected and clear in your mind, your body and heart will follow. The mind is the tool you wield to transform yourself. You can live a healthy and brilliant life if you just first start to imagine it. And expect it.

Look further into the future and believe that you will one day create something beyond what your imagination will even allow for this moment. The picture will change again and again. It will reveal more and more to you if you seek to know.

The ancient way of transformation is holistic. By holistic, we mean to recognize and approach all the parts that make up "the whole" person: the physical body, mental body, emotional body, soul, and spirit. This blueprint will take you through a series of stepping stones to get in touch with all of these parts to detox and cleanse all of you. We are going to identify where blockages occur, on all levels of body, mind, and heart. We'll set some life plans. Knowing all parts of yourself and how they all connect will help you to transform yourself, your health, and every other aspect that you wish to change. And it will demonstrate how everything that appears on the outside is an extension of what is going on in the inside. It is my vision and hope that you will get connected, get healed, live healthy, conscious, and exceptionally happy, forever. And when this great moment of triumph has occurred for you, pass the cup, share what you know so others can know as well, that the greatest story ever told says this: the Grail promises the right to restoration, regardless of what we have done in our life, to become whole again, complete, and perfect.

Cheers!

chapter 1

A Journey in Transformation

Wake-up Call

I've had my share of wake-up calls, like most people. A big one came in my early twenties. Immediately after graduating high school in 1978 I began to suffer stomach problems which included severe heartburn, nausea, cramping, and diarrhoea. Unfortunately, I ignored the symptoms for three years until it turned into an acute head-to-toe skin disease which appeared overnight.

I was finishing my third and final year of college studying architectural and interior design when my class flew to New York for an annual design show. Our chosen hotel was my first introduction to a world not so nice: rooms by the hour, a bullet-proof check-in counter, cockroach infestation (we slept with the lights on), and homeless people in the lobby. At night we met some seedy characters, some of whom I rubbed elbows with at the infamous nightclub Studio 54. (My professor would not have approved had she known!) Thinking back, whoever approved our hotel selection didn't do their homework.

Even though there were some scary, skin crawling moments on that poorly supervised trip, it was one more life experience that was quenching an insatiable thirst to know everything about this world. I feel fortunate in many ways to have acquired throughout my lifetime some fairly eye-opening, mind-bending, hair-raising, and head-shaking experiences, although many I would recognize now as dangerously irresponsible and even life-threatening. My friends and I have often reflected on how remarkably invincible we all felt in our youth. But that free-wheeling sense of immortality came to an abrupt halt in 1982. I became that "girl interrupted." For over twenty years in fact. It all began on this trip to New York.

During the short plane ride back I had an itch and noticed a tiny bump on the palm of my right hand. Unfortunately, it was not a sign that I was about to come into a pile of money. On the contrary, I was about to enter a trial by fire. Literally. I was about to feel like I was burning up on the outside of my skin.

A few days after arriving home the itching spread between my fingers, up the inside of my arms to my armpits, down my chest and around my waist. Soon I was covered from head to toe in this burning rash and within a week or so it was inside my mouth and groin. There wasn't a place that wasn't infected. The more I itched the worse it became. At the time I worked in a bar, and since I looked quite repulsive to bar patrons, my employers asked that I stay home until this eruption passed. This evening job was my only source of income, so I was soon unable to pay rent on time and got into trouble with my landlord.

It was a rough time. My parents had divorced a few years earlier. They sold the family home. Sadly, for a while I lost the close relationship I had had with my mother. Only in her mid-thirties then, she was going through her own life crisis and journey in self-discovery. I had no idea or care in the world what my younger and only brother Andrew was doing, and had lost all touch with any high school and neighbourhood friends.

I knew where my dad was, however. I was keeping a close eye on him. An off-and-on-again recovering alcoholic, he was also struggling through a very difficult time. By this time he had lost everything: first his driver's licence, then his wife, his home, the family, his car, his established career with a major brewery (which, as it turned out, saved his life). Eventually, he lost the little apartment condo he had purchased after the divorce. I found him a room in a boarding house close to the flat I was renting. He was destitute and suicidal on several occasions, almost succeeding the first time had I not found him in time.

He continued for another year to struggle with his addiction. My idea of helping was to steal the half-empty bottles out from under his bed when he was asleep and hope that he couldn't afford to buy another. We were living in a town often referred to as "the armpit of Ontario." I couldn't have agreed more, especially in my current state of mind. They say you are in the right place at the right time in your life. If that is true, it was clearly a reflection of how I was feeling towards life – the pits.

There was a pervert living next door who loved to do more than flash. I was terrified coming home late at night after work even after he was arrested. There were boyfriend troubles. My childhood dog died. My cats peed all over my roommate's art project one day. Granted, I had collected too many cats. Or more accurately, I couldn't give them up. The roommate was furious and moved out, which put me under more financial strain. One cat got lost for three weeks and then finally returned by some miracle, only to be hit and killed by a car days later. You get the picture. I was living Murphy's Law. More specifically, I was living the Law of Attraction big time.

My memory recalls my state of mind. I didn't care what was happening at that point in my life. I was angry with the world. There was arrogance and an attitude of "bring it on." But a good shot of humility came quickly. The skin condition became repulsive. And I was repulsive to myself, inside and out.

The burning was excruciating, especially at night. I covered myself with petroleum jelly and plastic wrap, wrapping myself up like an Egyptian mummy to ease the pain. Wearing pyjamas or sleeping with a bed sheet over my body was unbearable. Showering, washing my hair, or even brushing my teeth became impossible. And dressing — forget it. I eventually landed in the hands of a dermatologist who diagnosed it as lichen planus, a more common virus today, one for which they still know no cure. I can still feel the lesions leftover from the disease inside my mouth, a good reminder of where I've been, and to be grateful for my excellent state of health today. Doctors speculate that lichen planus may be contracted from cats. I've done animal rescue most of my life, so it was quite possible in my case that that was where I contracted the disease. Over the years, I've often joked about it though, laying blame on the cockroach-infested, room-by-the-hour hotel on 42nd Street where my journey began.

My skin specialist prescribed cortisone. I blew up like a balloon and the medication didn't work. In fact, my condition got worse. I was now in a wheelchair, as it became impossible for me to stand on my feet. My skin was cracking and bleeding from the soft orifices of my body. I was crying all the time. Depression was consuming me although I had no idea that's what it was.

The Acid Factor

Five weeks into my condition my mom, who had been frantic to find me help, called. A girlfriend of hers recommended we see a German herbalist she knew. Not wasting any time we were soon in the car travelling to a home outside of Toronto. I prayed he had a cure. He took me down into his basement office, sat me in a chair, looked into my eyes, checked my tongue, hands, and scalp. He tapped me here and there. In his thick German accent he said something that was going to play a huge role in my own vocation in assisting others in the future. He did not name the ailment. It did not matter to him. He said something about the acidic level in my body being extremely high. He went on to say that the root cause of my skin condition was an imbalance in my colon and intestines, and that the root cause of my colon imbalance was my diet. Most importantly too, he said there was an emotional imbalance.

No doubt my diet was at its worst. Anyone who has lived the college life knows the diet well: pop, coffee, beer, cigarettes, pot, speed pills, chocolate bars, doughnuts, macaroni and cheese, pizza and usually all of the above at 2:00 AM. I had been working at the bar most nights until 1:00 AM and then going to classes the next morning. Sleep deprivation didn't help matters. I started to clue in. At the root of my skin condition was my ongoing stomach problem. And at the root of my stomach problem, was not only diet but an emotional imbalance, to say the least. It was a "eureka" moment. My family – my mom, my dad, my brother and I – were all broken, and not just physically split apart; we were all broken in every which way, emotionally, mentally, and spiritually.

The herbalist pulled a series of wrinkled brown paper bags

with scribbled labels on them out of his dispensary. We went back upstairs to his kitchen where he boiled a big pot of water on the stove. He reached into each bag and pulled out handfuls what looked like bark and leaves from trees, peat-like substances, and mosses, tossed them into the pot and boiled it all together. Once it cooled down he strained it and had me drink a glass. The taste was not even close to being palatable, but I got it down. He sent me home with more of this alchemist's brew. Each night and each morning I was to boil same thick black potion, drink one glass and throw the rest into the tub and bathe in it. The itching stopped immediately. Within days my skin began to peel and new pink skin appeared. Within a week, I was well on my way to a complete recovery. I felt I was literally stepping from darkness and into the light.

This was my first personal experience with natural medicine and I started to clearly recognize the mind-body connection and its undeniable relationship to one's measure of health.

For me this was also a wake-up call about the disassociation the allopathic medicine world had with the naturopathic medicine world. I went back to the dermatologist with great excitement. I wanted to tell him about this miraculous cure so that he could share it with all his patients who might be suffering from the same ailment. Instead, I was asked to leave his office, but not before he chastised me and threw his pen across the room, barely missing my head and hitting the wall behind me. I left in shock, humiliated, and in tears. It took a lot of years for me to regain any trust in the allopathic world. Today, my circles of respected doctor friends are those who embrace the two worlds in their regular practice.

I ended up losing my college degree that year for not finishing. This was unfortunate because I was a good student and I know I would have gone far in the field I had chosen. For years I regretted this and felt it was a reflection of failure. What I eventually learned though, was that my appreciation for good design and skill for envisioning and creating beautiful spaces is innate. It's a passion that I have carried with me wherever I go, wherever I live, and with whatever I do. Little did I know that this passion for design and creating beautiful spaces would combine with my personal health crisis and manifest one day into one of the greatest projects of my life.

The Fear Factor

I continued to explore alternative therapies, taking courses, and even working for the Shiatsu School of Canada for a short time. I was still, however, suffering from a stomach disorder and problem bowel. I was told it was probably chronic. The stomach disorder lasted from 1979 to 2003. For eight of those years it became very difficult to leave the house for very long. If I went anywhere, it had to be a short journey and I had to plan a precise route, to the extent that I needed to know where every single gas station or public washroom was and even how much time there would be between stops. The problem perpetuated into anxiety attacks. More specifically, I had a fear of losing control of my bowels in public.

This fear had begun on a trip home from British Columbia in late 1979, also while on a flight. (It's no wonder I couldn't get myself on a plane for over a decade following all of this.) In the middle of one of these bowel attacks I was told I could not leave my seat because of the turbulence. You can imagine what happened next. I broke out in a profuse sweat, the world started to spin and then boom, I fainted in the middle of the aisle. After a few more experiences just like that one, I could no longer bear the thought of travelling. This led to having anxiety attacks over the thought of having anxiety attacks. It was crazy. But that's how it works. Your mind gets on the hamster wheel and you feel like there is no way off. My illness was infecting my mind and my mind was making me more ill. From my perspective now, fear is one of the most potent illnesses of all and I have made a vow to myself to continuously find and overcome anything at all inside of me that ever resembles fear. Fear almost killed me. I knew then that I needed to overcome myself, and my own mind, for healing to happen.

There were days I thought I would surely develop some horrible stomach disease, like cancer. I was convinced I would die young. Some days I would keel over with stomach spasms just from sipping water. My weight at times dropped to just over a hundred pounds and I was hospitalized more than once from dehydration caused by relentless diarrhoea. I quietly suspected that I could be suffering from Crohn's disease, ileitis, or colitis. Getting diagnosed seemed like the next obvious step to take. I had been warned by nurses and other health practitioners that if I didn't get this looked at and it continued, I could end up with a colostomy. A colostomy is a procedure in which an artificial opening is made from the colon through the abdominal wall which bypasses a diseased portion of the lower intestine. In other words, I'd have to wear a bag on the outside of my body for the rest of my life. When you are in your mid-twenties a solution such as this seems like a death sentence. I refused to get tested. I had a friend with Crohn's and another who had had a colostomy. I was afraid that if I allowed a diagnosis my fate would be sealed forever. The most I allowed for was testing positive and getting treated for parasites. The search for a different kind of cure continued.

Birth of The New Age

It was the '80s and many of you would remember it as the birth of the New Age movement. Toronto was saturated with New Age gurus, channelling demonstrations, prosperity workshops and conventions, self improvement seminars, motivational speakers, psychic shows, alternative therapy courses, crystal healing, tarot and pendulum readings, transcendental meditation, and so on. I admit I signed up for most of it. It fulfilled a curiosity mostly but it didn't have all the answers I needed to heal myself.

One day, in the latter part of the '80s, just before the new age movement as we knew it collapsed, I received a ticket to see the Dalai Lama at the University of Toronto. The audience was privy to a teaching being given to an inner group of disciples. We were allowed headphones and the lesson was translated into English. I didn't hear a word spoken, not a thing. I was deep in emotional and mental anguish. I could only look upon this group and wish for myself this elusive thing I was seeing called joy, calm, and peace of mind. I was feeling both reverence and grief at the same time. As our group descended from the lecture hall I could barely speak. I was distraught. I left the others to wander and wonder.

Ironically, in spite of not getting the lesson, it was a turning point in my life. I didn't connect with the spoken words, but I did connect with the essence of an alternative state of mind. A single life-changing thought was welling up inside my head. And here it was: that I had the undeniable right to achieve the same joy, calm, and peace of mind that they had; that I was not expected to renounce my life as I saw it – with a life partner, with children, and a design career. I was not expected to shave my head, wear a robe, or give up years of my life to study in a monastery away from the world I knew. I do have to admit though, the latter did cross my mind for a moment!

I recall feeling this sense of certainty many times since. Asking or praying for answers and guidance, I innately felt the universe was designed to give us answers. It was not to suppress or hide them, although I met many teachers along the path who did. Now the question for me was not "is it possible?" but rather "how do I access it?" So, I made it my quest to figure it out. I started with prayer, which really had become foreign to me, having not done so since I was much younger. Depending on how sincere I was in the asking, answers started to flow. I started to gain evidence of something greater at work here.

The '80s decade was somewhat revolutionary in that it introduced millions of individuals to the world of energies beyond the physical and universal intelligence as it relates to spiritualism. It freed many from religious dogma. There were growing pains. The New Age movement went out with a bang towards the end of the decade, mainly because it lacked the integrated science to support it and often lacked integrity. Too many hustlers looking for money clouded the vision. But it would be back another day, this time with more intelligence.

The '90s found people's interests drawn towards the "new age" of computer technology, the World Wide Web, world economics and foreign affairs, much of the latter stimulated by the Clinton era and the birth of CNN. It was an exciting time in politics. It was because of Bill Clinton, Hillary and the Gores that I, too, became much more globally minded and interested. Millions of people also aspired to expand their global view, while our planet seemed to contract and get smaller and smaller due to the new information highway and technology. It was a momentous time.

Today, in 2007, there is a resurgence of some of the New Age concepts, most stemming from ancient methods, but it is now paired with the science behind it. What is exciting is the coming together of the different fields of thoughts, including quantum physics and metaphysics. We can often see these two mediums sharing the same stage at science conventions, and in enlightening film documentaries such as *What the Bleep Do We Know?* and *The Secret*. Many scientists, visionaries, and spiritual teachers have come to acknowledge that there is very little separation between science and spiritualism. This is a great development in the evolution of human consciousness.

After that day with the Dalai Lama I was introduced to an ancient form of metaphysical study and mental yoga called Raja Yoga. This was the next monumental step in my healing process, which would take well over another decade. I immersed myself in Raja Yoga for eight years. I had a mentor and just like in a storybook I fell head over heals for my teacher, got married, and had my son Michael who is now ten years old. Though the union dissolved in 1999, I am grateful for what it brought. There was much happiness for a while, but it too was full of unending tests and challenges that my level of maturity at the time was not prepared for. Raja Yoga (the Grail Mantra on page 44 embodies the essence of ancient Raja Yoga) continues to be a guide to me and a method of self-discovery. It is a way of life and I have slowly come to introduce it in my lectures and classes at Grail Springs. It has allowed me access to understanding the way in which life and mind works, and has given me a clear path in which to walk the rest of my life. I owe my path, my present good health, and gratitude to both the teacher and the teaching.

Raising Grail Springs

There is a funny story behind the property now known as Grail Springs. For three years starting in 1990, my son's father and I searched for a place to start our life and build a bed and breakfast that would also serve as a place to hold retreats. We searched from California to Nova Scotia. What we didn't see was that the property was right under our noses, only a twenty minute drive north of Silent Lake, our favourite provincial campground. First we operated it with close friends as a bed and breakfast, holding small retreats. Then we opened the dining room up to the public and it created a whole new era that then led us into the wedding business. Talk about stress! We soon found ourselves operating as successful innkeepers but losing touch with our dreams to run a healing retreat centre. Finally in 2001 we made the decision to take the leap and add a spa segment, hoping it would allow us a way to get back to our roots and still generate a living. Grail Springs has undergone its own transformation many times over, and I expect it to continue, only to get better and better as the years go on.

When we first arrived, we discovered that the locals described the property as "The Kitchen Sink" because in its past it was everything but the kitchen sink. It had been a cattle farm, a local fishing hole, campground, laundromat, go-cart track, waterbed sales depot, and a used appliance sales and repair business. Dozens of old rusty appliances, tires, and parts scattered throughout the acreage had to be removed. Seeing past the immediate clutter it was clear to me that underneath it all, there was great hidden potential and beauty. A quiet sense of presence existed here, unlike my own inner voice that was screaming to "buy" and "buy today!" I thought I might hyperventilate if the paperwork wasn't signed as soon as possible.

The property consists of 100 acres of both hard- and softwood forest and trails and embraces a serene 50 acre spring-fed lake. It wasn't until a few years after we bought Grail Springs that I became aware of the unique alkaline properties of the water. Levels of acidity or alkalinity are determined by pH (pressure of hydrogen) levels. The state of typical water is neutral, or 7.0 pH. Vitamin C is about 4.5 on the acidic side of the pH scale. Baking soda is up around 10 on the alkaline side of the pH scale. We want mildly alkaline water, not acidic, as our bodies like to be more alkaline, the pH of the blood being 7.41. As Dr. Haas has described in the foreword, much disease may be linked to overly acidic lifestyles (acidic food and drink, acid-inducing stress). To maintain an alkaline state is a good path to health.

The land at Grail Springs is framed by a granite ridge that slopes up from the water's edge and beckons you into its forest. This is where my heart and home is today, on the edge of the forest. It's exactly where I wish to be in this life, living in-between the outer world of activity and creation and the still, inner world of calm and potential.

The Grail forest is alive today with abundant wildlife, a sign of a healthy environment. I have been drawn to the woods since being captured by the mystique of the Black Forest when I was seven years old. Hidden within the Grail forest are several special groves where I often go to contemplate, my secret hideaways.

Everyone should have a special place that calls to him or her. I envision this place as the very same as Arthur's vision of Camelot, a sanctuary where all people can flourish, heal, restore, and transform their lives. I am grateful to all those who laboriously helped to carve out and shape this beautiful place, and those friends and family members who supported the building of the Grail both financially and spiritually. Though I am now the sole proprietor, this place feels much more suited to a position of guardianship rather than ownership. It's a place to be shared with as many individuals as possible for its healing energy has become known to many as quite potent and effective.

Restoring Balance

As the years passed, and after I snapped out of two-and-a-half years in post-partum depression in 2000 after the birth of my son, my bouts with chronic diarrhoea were becoming noticeably fewer and fewer. In 2003, I was getting ready to design and integrate the first holistic detox cleanse program for Grail Springs. A friend in the entertainment industry introduced me to Sabra Ricci, a freelance celebrity chef based in Maui, who specialized in healthy cuisine catering to high profile individuals including top Fortune 500 CEOs and some of the biggest names in Hollywood. She had, over the years, versed herself in every type of diet on the market, designing gourmet meals around client's preferences. She's the gal to call when you need a special dining experience at your holiday villa, on your yacht or private jet, or when you need to get in shape for a film project. She has found her niche in the marketplace.

The first time we spoke on the phone I asked her this: if I were to introduce a prescribed diet at Grail Springs what would she recommend? Her answer was to look at the acid/alkaline approach to diet. That sounded vaguely familiar but I hadn't yet made the connection to my past. We quickly became friends and within weeks she flew out to Grail Springs where we spent an entire summer preparing and designing the program and menus along with a naturopathic doctor who had also recommended and supported the same diet. The three of us worked closely together and to my amazement my stomach was in complete agreement with everything that Sabra and I were churning out of our kitchen.

Today, I would absolutely insist upon the single realization that maintaining a proper pH balance in the body must become understood by the world as a major key to obtaining optimum wellness, weight management, and more specifically, disease prevention. Dr. Hass concurs with this, and he has had more than three decades of experience watching people shift to alkaline diet therapies and seeing how their various aches and pains go away. Their weight goes down, and their energy goes up. The good doctor also states that he believes in the "one disease" model – i.e. cellular dysfunction leads to a great variety of health problems. There are two cause of disease, as Dr. Haas alludes to in the foreword: one is a deficiency of the necessary and vital nutrients that we get from fresh and wholesome foods (which allow our cells to perform the myriad range of functions they do every second of every day.) The other is toxicity that comes from chemical and metal exposures or imbalanced diets that affect the enzymes and cell functions.

I can't say enough about the acid/alkaline approach to diet and what we ourselves have witnessed here at Grail Springs for the past four years. It is astounding how quickly the body responds and heals when it is given the right biochemical or nutritional balance to work with. The pH balance approach to diet, along with six other elements, have become the foundation and contributed to the success of the Grail Springs programs. Good health, joy, peace of mind, and longevity can all happen when there is balance in your body and in your life.

chapter 2

Seek, Find, and Drink from the Cup

The Grail Code

Mysteries, dynasties, adventures, and noble knights, these are the impressions that come to mind when one hears "The Grail." It has been sought after throughout time and history, and it is believed that its divine powers hold the gift of healing, enlightenment, and even eternal life. It is said that this can be had by any who seek, find, and drink from the cup itself.

Grail Springs was the very first impression that came to mind when it was time to choose a name for the wellness centre, as the lake bubbled with fresh spring water from the ancient granite bedrock below.

Because I had been intrigued by the legends of the Holy Grail for years – stories of Merlin, King Arthur, Excalibur and the Lady of the Lake   the cup was undoubtedly the perfect choice, the ultimate global icon, a symbol of hope for all who seek to be whole. The mystery of the Grail's continued popularity century after century may lie in the fact that the essential values it represents are those most people thirst for: to be good, to be true, and to be happy.

The ancient Grail Code, "Ich Diene," was born from the Age of Chivalry and translates from German to English as "I serve." It is this ancient code which we have adopted into our work here at Grail Springs. The chalice supports the ideal of service to mankind, and the fluid content corresponds to the spirit of fulfillment and restoration. This would be one of many interpretations. When the name appeared, it was an easy choice to make.

Goddess of Truth, Justice & Forgiveness

The Grail tradition goes as far back as Mesopotamia, an area now recognized as the southern regions of Iraq. It was here that astronomy, alchemy, an education system, and medicine were developed and supported. In Ur, one of the world's first flourishing cities, a social structure and philosophy called "Maat" began. Ancient Egyptian text translates it as "Goddess of Truth and

Justice." The teachings were lost for thousands and thousands of years. Joseph of Arimathea is said to be the first member of the Grail families to restore the old traditions, around A.D. 6. Joseph is associated with the most common image, the cup that captured the blood of Jesus, also said to be the cup of the Last Supper. Some legends have it that Mary Magdalene, Simon, and other remaining family members and disciples sailed to the South of France while Joseph, who remained in possession of the cup, moved even farther north to spread the word of truth. What stands today as the ruins of Glastonbury Abbey, a three-hour drive from London, England, is said to be the very site where Joseph of Arimathea built the first Christian Church and here protected the Grail cup. Thousands upon thousands of individuals visit this site every year. It is also said to be the burial site of King Arthur and his Queen Guinevere.

I finally made my first visit to Glastonbury this past summer of 2007 and also visited the famous healing waters of the Chalice Well. My quest was twofold. In many ways it was a grail quest of the old tradition, to fill my cup, to seek, contemplate and find more truth, meaning, and inspiration for the next chapter of my life. And it was also to lay to rest the ashes of one of my dearest friends who lost her battle with breast cancer the previous year. Chandra regarded Glastonbury as one of her favourite places on earth aside from Grail Springs. She felt most connected there, and so this trip was all the more meaningful.

As I sat in the gardens of the Chalice Well, I reflected on all the historic legends and personalities of Grail lore and traditions. I thought of Chandra, who only a couple of years before me had sat quietly in meditation in this same garden. The cancer seeds in her body would have already been active though not yet discovered. If she were alive today she would tell you that these seeds were planted decades earlier from living an unhealthy lifestyle. She was of a generation that didn't yet understand the consequences of smoking, drugs, and alcohol. A carefree flower child living through the free-loving '60s and a fantastic singer, she landed a dream job as the booking co-ordinator for the famous Troubadour Club in West Hollywood. Her life got off track, and in her late thirties she tried to turn things around. She spent the last couple of decades living in and around Chicago dedicating many of those years working in a temple as a student of yoga. She loved her guru and gave it her all to fix some of the things she had broken in her life. But she still struggled with regret right to the end. It consumed her heart and mind. She quietly hoped for acceptance and forgiveness from some of her children. It didn't come in the end the way she had envisioned it and that was painful to see. I thought it insensitive and unjust, but also understood it as the plight of our human condition sometimes.

Part of our message at Grail Springs is to forgive everyone in your life who you think has crossed you. There is no resolve or peace or restoration possible while you hold them hostage, for them or for us. Set them free from blame. Your parents and children have their own passage in life. They too have suffered and felt their own loss and have been broken. They too have the right to restoration and peace as every one of us does.

Guardians of The Grail

A few centuries after Joseph of Arimathea, Roman Emperor Constantine intervened and brought about the system known today as Catholicism. The Grail teachings of truth and justice became a mystery once more, remaining buried for several centuries, though not all was lost. By the sixth century the Grail families had grown and spread throughout Europe. The need to protect the families as well as the secrets of the Grail was recognized and measures were taken. Many monastic orders of the era followed a lifestyle separate from the episcopacy of the Roman Church, and often hid their beliefs within their beautiful manuscripts, using watermarks and secret codes. Even the Tarot pack has intimate connections with hidden Grail traditions.

In the early eleventh century, guardianship of the Grail was adopted by a group of knights, warrior monks who served the Crusades calling themselves The Knights Templar, the forerunners of the Rosicrucians and Freemasons. They quickly became very powerful. One of their mandates was to protect Christian pilgrims who were en route to Jerusalem, considered the Holy City of God at the time. These men took vows of poverty, chastity, and obedience, and were renowned for their loyalty and courage in battle.

Over recent decades there have been hundreds of researchers, academics, archaeologists, and authors uncovering and rewriting the history of the Grail. In such bestselling books as *Holy Blood, Holy Grail*, published in 1983, and the blockbuster novel *The Da Vinci Code*, it is suggested that there is some evidence Jesus and Magdalene were united as husband and wife with several children of their own. Magdalene and her entourage were thought to have sailed to the South of France, embraced and aided by the people of the land. It is also thought that Magdalene and other female apostles brought about the first hospices to heal the sick and teach the secrets of alchemy, herbal medicine, and other energy healing therapies. Science, music, art, literature, and Grail dynasties such as the French Merovingian began to flourish. Education was encouraged and women were considered equal in every regard.

The Cathars were one such community who kept alive the knowledge of the Grail, but in the thirteenth century met their demise on the famous site of Montsegur by orders of the Pope. There are many streets, chapels and icons representing the presence of this group in modern-day Montsegur. Communities were built, sites and monuments were erected where they say the secrets of the Grail and scrolls from the Temple of Solomon were re-deposited and later adopted and protected by the infamous Knights Templar. The Knights Templar are very much responsible for protecting many of the healing traditions and bringing to our minds today such tools as the amazing sacred Labyrinth, which we will explore in a later chapter.

The Pursuit of Happiness

Wherever secret codes and hidden treasures exist, legends and folklore will blossom. The most famous is the legend of King Arthur, Camelot, and the Knights of the Round Table, my favourite story of all. Arthur and his Knights painstakingly learn that the Grail is not a golden treasure to be possessed, but rather a journey in self-discovery and restoration. By becoming of pure heart and pure mind one is rewarded with the secrets of the Grail, the secrets of life ever after.

After breaking free from Roman control in the late fifth century and moving to the north, Arthur, a respected commander in the army, had a vision. He was going to build the perfect world. He knew that even his Knights, who for most of their lives had known only a life of brutality, were at their heart good men, and that they too had the right to redeem themselves and live a life of peace and productivity. He saw a world free from war and battle, pain and suffering. He vowed to build a city where all citizens could flourish, where all men and women were equal and who were endowed by their Creator with the right to pursue life, liberty, and happiness. If this sounds familiar, it is because it is the founding idealism for America's Declaration of Independence. It is known that some of the delegates who wrote it in 1776 were indeed Masons; most prominent among them, Thomas Jefferson and Benjamin Franklin.

You may recall this story being shown on the big screen if you saw the 2005 adventure movie starring Nicolas Cage called *National Treasure*. It was about a man who was obsessed with finding the legendary Knights Templar treasures but has to decipher ancient riddles one after another that will lead him to the hidden burial chamber. He has to borrow (steal) the Declaration of Independence for a while, as it contains one of the pieces of the puzzle. Naturally, I was first in line upon its release both because of my Grail interest but also because I happen to be a huge Nicolas Cage fan. After the movie, I had always thought that I would love to meet Cage one day and see if the making of this film had an impact on his life. Did it pique his curiosity about finding the true meaning of the Grail?

Here's a great bit of trivia for you and evidence to me that the universe is always responding to your thoughts. I collect Grail cups, and I was projecting that on this trip to Arthurian land, I would discover "the" cup, something really significant that I could bring home to my collection. While staying at the sweetest bed and breakfast called Hotel No. 3 on Magdalene Avenue, on what was once part of the Glastonbury Abbey grounds, my son and I would look forward each morning to a gorgeous breakfast in the parlour room where we would also meet up with the other Grail pilgrims and hear their fabulous stories of discoveries from the day before. We were led on some terrific journeys each day as a result of this morning session, including to a fresh crop circle and the hidden location of ancient Camelot.

My son and I became instant friends with a couple from Vermont who specialize in the manufacturing and distribution of gems and gem jewellery world wide. We didn't know it, but we had landed in Glastonbury just when the town was gearing up for the International Crystal & Sound Conference. Robert Simmons was there as a guest speaker, an author and expert in his field who has written several books on gems. One book in particular is *Moldavite: Starborn Stone of Transformation*. I had never heard of this stone, which I thought unusual since I have been surrounded for years by healers who use crystals and gems in their work. I had read of the Grail stone and the Philosopher's stone, but had never read any reference to what it actually was. Many historians believe that the references to this stone "that fell from the sky" is Moldavite. Moldavite is a gem that fell to earth, in the region of Czechoslovakia some 14 million years ago and has been used by humans as talismans for over 25,000 years.

That very day was the day we had planned to visit the gardens of the Chalice Well to scatter Chandra's ashes. On our way out we visited the gift shop where we found many wonderful books and treasures. But the greatest treasure of all did not capture my attention until I was at the cash desk tallying up, and I looked in a glass case to my left. There was a most delicate hand-blown green glass cup, and it was clearly calling out to me. The lovely gentleman serving me brought the cup out for me to handle. I didn't notice at first, but eventually I saw five green stones embedded around the outside of the vessel. I asked what they were and you can guess what he said; "It is Moldavite." I was stunned and of course without hesitation told him this cup was meant for me. Well, the story doesn't end here. As he was wrapping up the cup, he told me I might like to know another little piece of information to add to the whole mystique of my finding this cup that day. He said that the cup had a sister cup, and that it had just been purchased weeks before me by another visitor to the Chalice Well. And that someone was none other than Nicolas Cage. It was a happy day.

[
The Ancient Grail Code:
"*Ich Diene*" translates from German
to English as "I Serve."
]

The Promise of Restoration

The first mention of Arthur's "Round Table" was in Wace's *Roman de Brut*. It was said to have seated fifty knights and its round shape suggested equality among all. The stories of the Knights of the Round Table reflected the ideals of the chivalric code "I Serve," and the court of King Arthur became the centre of order, justice, and civility. It was the first time a king sat side by side with council.

Arthur shared a further idealism with council. No decision would be acted upon until a unanimous vote was had – not a majority, but unanimous. He believed in the concept of a supreme truth. He argued that if each Knight could achieve a purified heart and a pure mind of objectivity, they would all then have the eyes to see and the ears to hear the absolute. They would reach unanimous agreement and it would be without a doubt the right action for all concerned.

Legend has it that Arthur built his Camelot. And his Knights once again took an oath in the spirit of "one for all and all for one," the famous charge adopted by the Three Musketeers. It was an oath of loyalty, to speak only in truth, to keep a virtuous heart, and to defend the innocent. It was by striving to live by this oath with all their might that the Knights of the Round Table sought restoration. They sought to redeem their heart, mind, body, and spirit. Standing in the light of the Great Hall in Camelot, the Cup of the Grail appeared to them, as an ethereal vision, pouring all of life's secrets onto them. Today we have the beautiful and mystical stories and legends that rose out of this command for healing, restoration, redemption, and even life ever after. It is said that the Grail avails itself to everyone. Its promise is that everyone has the right to restoration. You only have to seek it.

chapter 3
The Mind-Body Connection

What is Wellness?

The terms wellness and illness are a measurement of our "state" – of mind, emotions, and body. This state is in a constant flow, moving from one end of a spectrum to the other and measured moment by moment. Wellness and illness, one or the other, is happening at all times whether you know it or not, whether you are paying attention to it or not. This continuum is the process that each and every living organism, big and small, from a cellular level to plant, animal, human and even planetary, is going through from conception to death. It's a measurement of our state of being in-between these two points. Its range of potential would run from high level wellness at one end to premature death at the other end, with neutral being in the middle. You might ask yourself, where do you fall on the graph at this present time in your life? Where were you on the graph at other times in your life? And more importantly, where would you like to be now and into your future?

Illness-Wellness Continuum

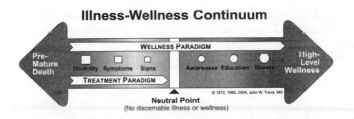

Moving from the centre to the left shows a progressively worsening state of health. Moving to the right of center indicates increasing levels of health and wellbeing. The treatment paradigm (drugs, herbs, surgery, psychotherapy, acupuncture, and so on) can bring you up to the neutral point, where the symptoms of disease have been alleviated. The wellness paradigm, which can be utilized at any point on the continuum, helps you move toward higher levels of wellness.

The wellness paradigm directs you beyond the neutral point and encourages you to move as far to the right as possible. It is not meant to replace the treatment paradigm on the left side of the continuum, but to work in harmony with it. If you are ill, then treatment is important, but don't stop at the neutral point. Use the wellness paradigm to move toward high-level wellness.

It helps to clearly know where you are at in order to know where you are going. Developing a life plan is a key to your success. A regular self maintenance check on your state of health mentally, emotionally, and physically is recommended often. Because I have experienced both ends of the illness-wellness spectrum I have become sensitive to how I am feeling moment to moment. If my chemistry is off, I notice right away. A quick read comes to mind when I feel strong and also when I feel depleted. I don't let myself get too far off-centre without acting on it. It is amazing how quickly the body will balance itself out with just a little attention. If I feel a flu bug coming on, I get myself into an Austrian moor mud bath and take a variety of extra supplements of some kind. This is the fine-tuning that I try to teach people to be aware of.

In the beginning, it can take months to connect all the dots. It depends where you are at on the illness-wellness continuum. If you find yourself on the right side of the continuum, you've more than likely already done some work and are aware of what it takes to maintain it. If you think you are on the left side of the scale, congratulations on picking up this book. You have just made the first step to turning things around.

At the Heart of the Matter

Our emotional state seems the easiest to identify in ourselves and others because it appears in real time through the actions we or others express. We identify it quickly by our feelings or moods. Emotions like laughter and joy can be uplifting and healing, while emotions like fear or bitterness can be toxic and destructive.

When you get angry or depressed it affects the nervous system's chemistry and weakens the immune system. Emotional memories are stored and bound to the nervous system until they are understood and released. They also affect people's digestive tract, or whatever their weak areas are. The visual memory is stored in the occipital cortex of the brain (back of the head). Ancient healing practices suggest that there are certain emotions that inherently find their place in the nervous system of specific organs. For example, Chinese medicine observes the autonomic nervous system, which has an effect on the heart rate, digestion, respiration rate, salivation, and perspiration. This energy is also thought to travel through specific pathways beneath the skin's surface, called meridians to and through the organs. When negative emotions are experienced, there is either an overabundance of energy, a depletion of energy, or it gets blocked altogether, and this has an effect on the illness-wellness continuum of the organs themselves.

An example of the correlation between emotions and organs from ancient Chinese practices:

Emotion	Organ
Worry	Lung, stomach
Fear	Kidneys, bladder
Anger	Gall bladder, liver
Grief	Pancreas, spleen, colon, lungs
Lack of acceptance/ sadness	Heart, small intestine
Guilt	Upper back, lungs
Financial burden/ lack of support	Lower back

You have to know where you are at on the path to know where you are going.

What is not always so noticeable is the actual state of illness our body is in until the first sign of trouble appears. Physical matter is much slower to manifest than emotions. In traditional Chinese medicine, all health issues have an energetic basis before there is a physical symptom or sign of disease. Some chronic problems may come from decades of imbalance.

Until an illness reaches an acute situation, most of us are not aware of the gradual process as it is happening. If our stress level is rising for some time, signs like general weakness, irritability, fatigue, headaches, and constipation can be early indications that the flow of nutrients, oxygen and energy is being hindered.

Emotions such as grief and heartbreak can cause premature death. Hurricane Katrina devastated New Orleans on August 29th, 2005. The head of New Orleans' Health Department reported in June, 2006 that the state's death rate of 14.3 per 1,000 people during the first three months of 2006 topped the national mortality rate of 8.1 per 1,000 people. Citizens of New Orleans were still dying from cardiac conditions five months after the storm hit the city. Dr. Mehmet Oz, an accomplished and respected cardiovascular surgeon in the United States and regular consulting doctor on the Oprah Winfrey show, predicted that death due to cardiac failure was going to significantly rise in the immediate aftermath of the storm. He was right. The root cause he says, "was broken hearts," or "grief." Deep feelings of sorrow, pain and loss put a physical strain on the heart. They can also stress and weaken the immune system. The heart functions abnormally and creates the physical sensation of pain in the chest. Too much of this continued stress can prompt a heart attack. It's true; people can die of a broken heart.

Toxic Thoughts

In the 2006 documentary film *The Secret*, one of the guest speakers in the film, Mike Dooley, says it best, "thoughts become things." Our mental state is not always a topic we are prepared to talk about openly or easily. Generally we do not like to have our true state of mind exposed. ("If only they knew what I really thought.") Many people go out of their way to hide a mental condition like post-partum depression as if in shame, as I did. I could not even bring myself to tell anyone or to seek professional help. As recently as 2006, actress Brooke Shields took a brave step in exposing this dark secret that millions of mothers live through alone in her bestselling book *Down Came the Rain: My Journey Through Postpartum Depression*. Only then was there finally more open discussion about this syndrome. Let's face it, taking a good look at our state of mind can be an uncomfortable proposition for the average person, but it's good for our health.

How we spend our time thinking about life is how we are going to feel about life from moment to moment. This in turn has an immediate effect on the inner functions of the body like the nervous system, respiratory system, chemistry and energy. When the energy channels between the brain and the cells in an organ get plugged or impaired due to stress, the signal from the brain does not get to the cells in that organ with the command to empty the waste product. A cell containing energy or biochemical waste gets toxic and swells, causing the organ to stop functioning optimally. All kinds of deadly diseases can be caused when an organ's

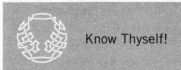

Know Thyself!

[
"Thoughts become Things"
–Mike Dooley, *The Secret*
]

function is weakened from the loss of brain signal. What appears as a mental or emotional imbalance can eventually make its physical appearance in our body as an ailment as a result. This is why we accept the idea today that stress and negative thinking can cause premature death.

As you begin to explore the connection between thought, emotions, and body, attempt to objectively investigate your state of health for the purposes of self-realization and growth. Where would you like to be on the illness-wellness continuum? Would you be happy living in the neutral zone or would you like to shoot for that "high level wellness."

Being responsible for your own health is a choice. It is only when you have chosen that your quest and journey for optimum health can begin, and not a moment before. Have courage. Once you get over the first hurdle or two, it becomes a ride of a different kind!

Cells vs. Toxins

Your body is a battlefield. Your cells are defending themselves against toxins every single moment. Toxins are poisonous substances that vary in their severity. Snake venom, for instance, is a toxin. But toxins can also exist in seemingly harmless plants, common foods, and in many of our daily household items. They can be ingested, absorbed by the skin, inhaled, and even produced by the body. Toxins interact with the cells' receptors, the channels which feed the cells. Where toxins build up, adverse reactions may occur, some of them serious. Where there is disease present, the natural cellular environment has in some way been disturbed, or altered, and an overburden of toxins will be present.

The effects can range from a simple skin rash or irritation, to swelling and inflammation, digestive problems like bloating, to major diseases, such as cancer. Toxins are everywhere in our daily life, from pollution in the air we breathe and the water we drink, to the preservatives and environmental chemicals in foods, and from excessive refined sugars and animal fats, or from highly processed junk foods. Toxins are also consumed when we smoke, drink alcohol excessively, and take pharmaceutical drugs.

Our cells live the same illness-wellness continuum that we do. Cells can thrive and live a healthy life or they can die a premature death just like us. Cells need energy in the form of nourishment, hydration and oxygen which is supplied to them by the surrounding fluids, mostly made up of water. Cells will take what they need by way of minerals and nutrients, and either transform it into energy or store it away for future use. The rest becomes waste, which they need to expel back into the surrounding fluids to be flushed away. This makes the composition of the surrounding interstitial fluids most important to your cellular health. If there is an overabundance of toxins and acids in the fluids it can alter the cells' ability to function and can ultimately change the cells' characteristics. If the cell isn't able to expel the waste, it swells. In other words, cells get constipated and congested just as we do. Cells are taking a bath every day in the surrounding fluids which either feed them the necessary nutrients and oxygen, or dehydrates them, leaving cells malnourished, bloated and unable to expel the waste. Sound familiar?

How we think and feel about life has a major influence on the state of our health.

Cells depend on:

- Right food
- Plenty of water, and the right amount of water so as not to dilute the minerals in your system
- Right exercise (keep the fluids and lymph system moving)
- Right environment
- Clear communication path

So we know that toxins are threatening to our cellular life. The trick is to not willingly consume foods and other substances that work against us, but rather choose to eat right in order to keep our cellular environment clean. And most importantly, we need to keep the fluids moving and flushing them out with exercise. This will keep toxins from creating an environment where they can take hold and do damage. Also, our lymphatic system, which helps to clear wastes from the body, does not have a pump like the heart and thus depends on exercise to provide that effective pumping and cleansing action.

A regular detoxifying body cleanse integrated into your lifestyle plan is an excellent form of defence against disease and a means of maintaining your overall good health. A detox program can consist of a one-week plan at the beginning of each season, whereby you give your body's digestive system a break. You might eliminate alcohol, caffeine, baked goods, dairy foods, and red meat, and instead revert to lighter fare, or a vegetarian or raw diet. Some of our detox plans at Grail Springs integrate a juice fasting program as well. Light exercise such as walking and

Everything depends on the health of our cells!

getting lots of fresh air, and Himalayan salt baths to help flush out the toxins and replenish your body with necessary minerals to start detoxifying your body.

Energy
The Language of the Universe

You are matter, you are light, and you are energy, eternally transforming yourself. Energy cannot be created or destroyed, but it can change forms. Every bit of matter in this universe can be broken. It can either be in a state of stored energy (potential), or kinetic energy (moving). Just like our cells, we can take energy in, we can store it, and we can spend it. We can be depleted of it or have too much of it at any one moment. It can get stuck with nowhere to go.

Energy in ⟶ Energy transformed ⟶ Energy out

Our bodies collect energy from available sources such as food, supplements, oxygen, and water, which our body transforms into mechanical energy, which is then used to help us move and get our work done. Solar energy is transformed into heat energy to keep our bodies warm and regulated. We also get energy from the environment or when we are doing something we love. We even get energy from what we call "vibes" from other people. All of the above can add to a higher level of wellness.

[
It is essential to take in equal amounts of energy to what you are expressing. Definition of "Burn Out": when you are expressing more energy out than you are taking in.
]

As above...

so below!
What happens in the mind affects our body and vice versa

On the other hand, exposure to energy can also make us ill if it's too much or if it's negative energy. We've often heard ourselves or friends saying how drained we feel when in the presence of a negative personality. Or when we are not doing what we love, when we don't eat the right foods, when we drink low energy substances such as alcohol, or when we get too much sun. The goal here is to tune into the language of the universe; energy. Everything has a frequency. Ask yourself, is this piece of food, this person, or the job that you are doing adding to your reserve or taking away from your reserve of energy? Am I getting enough sleep to recharge my body's batteries? Be sure your energy reserve is kept full and balanced in order to maintain optimum levels of energy.

Explore your world inside and out from an energetic perspective. It's how the entire universe converses and responds. Start asking yourself, "Is that which I am about to ingest going to serve my energy reserve or reduce it?"

The Bio-Energy Field

You have a "frequency." Your level of energy, and your level of vitality can be captured on film. It's called the bio-energy field and it is the total read of the life-energy or vitality of an organism. It surrounds every single living thing, a human being, an animal, a tree, a leaf, or a cell. Science has found a way to read these frequencies as they appear by way of a light and colour spectrum resulting from bio-feedback measurements.

Bio-feedback technology can capture what is h a p p e n i n g inside of us. It is

> We are all built from two components: biochemical matter and energy.

a picture of our overall vital energy, sometimes describes as our "vital body." In old world paintings you often see halos or auras painted around subjects. The aura is not a mysterious and mystical thing, it is simply the energetic picture of our body's state of wellness or illness. Today bio-feedback technology can be used to see imbalances both on a physical and mental level. It can take an accumulative read on the health of your chakras, your meridians and your organs.

This science originated as Kirlian photography, which came out of Russia in the 1930s, the first to capture this energy field. This photographic phenomenon happened by accident when Semyon Kirlian was exposed to a harmless electron cascade. He saw a visible aura around his hands which he captured on film. Based on Kirlian photography, scientists developed a theory that perhaps a stream of sub-atomic particles move in and out of living tissue which reveal important information about the life and health of an organism. Thanks to today's computer technology you can view a full moving bio-energy field in real time as it is receiving, transforming, and expressing energy.

Everything that appears in the physical body is reflected in its energy field and vice versa. Returning the flow of energy to normal is reflected in the field. Restoration and balance between the biochemical and bio-energy components can result in improved health. Ancient practices that work with the energy field have

Find your balance by tuning in to the language of the Universe, ENERGY!

reappeared in modern forms, such as Reiki, chakra balancing, craniosacral therapy, gem therapy, therapeutic touch, and the use of tuning forks, all of which bring balance to the bioenergetic flow and field of the body.

Seven Major Chakra Centres

Teachings in the ancient art of energetic healing encompass the practice of balancing and restoring the body's energy force, known by different cultures or practices as life-force energy, ch'i, prana, and vital or universal energy. When this energy is allowed to flow freely, it can enter from the top of the head and even in through the eyes and channel itself down and up along the spine, and outward through an alignment of seven major energy centres known as chakras. Chakra is a Sanskrit word which means "wheel." Each chakra exists as a swirling vortex of light and colour, a vibration if you will, forming a vacuum in the centre. This magnetic draw attracts to them anything that corresponds to their particular colour and light frequency spectrum.

The seven major chakras correspond to seven major organs and seven glands. There are an additional twenty-one secondary or minor chakras, each corresponding to different areas of the body. The workings of the chakra system are complex. There is a corresponding force for each of the seven major centres. It is through the process of evolution of consciousness that the energy forces to and from the chakras can be transferred and transmuted. Holistic health practitioners today use the foundation of ancient energy therapies to assist with balancing the chakra system in order to keep the free flow of life-force energy moving to the corresponding organs and glands.

 It's all about being in the right frequency!

Life energy will gather where your
consciousness is focused.

Again, how you think, feel and express yourself in this life
has an energetic effect on your physical vitality. Keeping your
chakras healthy and in balance by learning to quickly transform
your stress and negative thinking through meditation is an
approach that can be learned. A holistic therapy specifically
called "chakra balancing" is becoming more available as a means
to de-stress and keep the centres in balance. Yoga, breath work,
and meditation are all excellent ways to relax the body and
transform stress. It is encouraged to keep this energy flowing
and uninterrupted.

	Chakras	Colour	Glands	Organs
7th	Crown	White/Gold	Pineal	All
6th	Third Eye	Indigo	Pituitary	Brain
5th	Throat	Turquoise	Thyroid	Larynx
4th	Heart	Green	Thymus	Spleen
3rd	Solar Plexus	Yellow	Pancreas	Stomach
2nd	Sacral	Orange	Adrenal	Kidney
1st	Base	Red	Gonads	Sex Organs

Each of the seven major chakras represents seven states of consciousness as well. Let's look at animals for a moment. Their lower
chakras are most enlivened hence the dominating instinctual
nature, otherwise known as "animal instincts." These are survival

based and are mainly the first through the third charkas. For humans, chakras 4, 5, and 6 are the most dominant in the building and maintenance of our vital force. We live in a particular time in evolution in which we are more developed emotionally, mentally, creatively, and spiritually than ever before. We are communicators. We are more in control of our animal nature than might have been the case 30,000 years ago. You might say we are climbing the chakra scale as time goes on. This is also true in our life experience. As we move from birth to full adulthood, we have the potential to become more in control of our lower nature. As we age we develop our will and gain more self-control.

The individual who expresses an imbalance emotionally and mentally and doesn't take care of his or her physical needs will not be as open a receptor for downloading the life-force energy. They will find themselves drained and fatigued on every level and eventually could succumb to illness. When we are knocked out physically, our emotions are usually running rampant. We are irritable and sometimes even irrational in our thinking. As you become more balanced in your lifestyle choices, emotions, and thinking, you will be that much more receptive to drawing down the life-force energy, allowing it to move freely to "feed" you.

Universal Tree of Life

As we gain control of our negative urges we gain control of our power to utilize energy to add to our life, our creativity, our health, and our self-realization. Students of Buddhism, Raja Yoga or many other spiritual schools of thought will make it their goal to open the seventh Chakra in their lifetime. This is also known as the thousand-petalled lotus, the spiritual aspect of Self. Ancient teachings say that as the seventh Chakra opens, as the lotus unfolds, "spiritual" life-force pours in, allowing clearer and clearer access to something called "the Universal Tree of Life." The Tree of Life is the foundation of almost every ancient culture, from the Mayans and Aztecs, to the Nordics, to Kabbalists and Buddhists.

The roots of the tree represent human life, the physical realm, and the experience of earthly matters, while the branches and leaves represent the spiritual and cosmic realities. The trunk contains the heart and soul which connects the two worlds together. It is along the pathways through the trunk of the tree that information is passed and perceived by both roots and branches. Like the Celts who created the symbolic woven Celtic knot, we have the potential to learn how to weave and braid these two realities – heaven and earth – together, beautifully, masterfully, into our waking human life. That is a definition of an accomplished and perfect life. I think this is the same vision that King Arthur tapped into for his dream of Camelot and his Knights of the Round Table.

What is Soul?

The soul is light. Light is electromagnetic energy. It is a force. And it is coloured by a particular vibration or frequency of energy. The soul is the glue, the force holding together the world of matter and spirit. In Raja Yoga, the term "the light of the soul" is a perceived measurement of the quality and vitality of each person's soul and its outwardly expressed attributes. The more attributes an individual is embodying and expressing, the "brighter their light." We may not see the light with the naked eye, but we have often used this term to compliment someone who exudes many admirable traits such as kindness, compassion, playfulness, and joyfulness.

The seven major energy centres in your body are nourished by light energy – soul to soul energy!

Living life fully awake is our aim. There are many teachings and tools one can do to get into this flow of life. One technique I created by pure accident one day, is something we have implemented at Grail Springs called the World Mantra. I start every day of my life with the World Mantra. It is powerful in stirring up these soul attributes. It uses music, movement, and mindfulness through a moment of silence first, then a series of invocations, using specific words, such as "grace" and "gratitude."

Other suggested words for the World Mantra: Peace, Joy, Courage, Justice, Purity, Innocence, Benevolence

The World Mantra creates a specific rhythm within heart and mind, eventuates the essence of our potential, and our soul attributes rise to the surface. It usually stuns people the very first time they try this exercise. But it takes practice like anything else to make it permanent. It's like working out and trying to get your body in shape. The more you practice the stronger you get. There are daily tests and challenges. Sometimes you breeze through your day and sometimes you know you were unprepared or just didn't do what you said you would do out of laziness. One thing is guaranteed, you will most definitely get another chance. In fact, you get the rest of your life and many more lessons to keep figuring it out. You can take all the time you need.

The Grail World Mantra

Gratitude, humility, grace, and reverence, are all words that I have come to know as the language and expressions of the soul. These descriptive words and others like them are keys to unlocking the secrets of the seemingly elusive soul, connecting you directly with the source of all attributes that lay within you.

Invoking these words ignites the light of the soul within. As this source of electromagnetic energy fires and increases, its impressions are felt both by the individual and by those around as feelings (energy) emanating from the centre of their heart chakra. A powerful invocation like The Grail World Mantra activates and releases the energy not only in the heart chakra but also the throat chakra and the head chakra. This practice activates a process in which you find your place between the subconscious and the super conscious, a monumental moment in an individual's path of spiritual evolution. This is often referred to in different esoteric schools as "the awakening."

This practice feeds the whole of you: body, heart, mind, soul, and spirit. It was this single self-induced experience that snapped me out of two-and-a-half years of post-partum depression and gave me the inspiration to create a practice that could assist others. Today it has now become much more; an integral part of my continuous journey in self-discovery.

It began one morning in 1999. I was in the bathroom and had turned on the radio. Having just showered, I was standing naked, in more ways than one, in front the mirror. I was now a single mom, exhausted, overweight and out of shape, depressed, isolated, and feeling purposeless. I had not sought any professional help for my condition, and could not find a way to express my grief to anyone, not even my closest friends. But I was asking for help internally. I desperately wanted to find my way out of this darkness.

On this particular day, the theme song from the blockbuster movie Titanic; "My Heart Will Go On" came on the radio. Celine Dion's ethereal voice filled the room. I closed my eyes and just let the music pull me into some other place. I found myself standing tall, raising my arms up over my head and I just started to move into a standing yoga pose and then another. I hadn't done any movement in over three years. I felt like I was literally being lifted up by an unseen force. I could feel the presence of grace all around me. I was filling up with so much emotion it hurt. I hadn't felt anything in a very long time. By the end of the song I was on my knees, bawling with bittersweet joy and gratitude. I was stunned by what had just happened. I knew that I had just been completely released from my depression. I haven't had a day of depression since, and I begin every day of my life with this World Mantra, incorporating my Raja yoga practise into the routine. Over the past few years I've had the absolute pleasure of sharing the World Mantra with thousands of individuals at Grail Springs.

You can set it to any music that moves you. I most often use Deva Premal's "Aad Guray." Both Celine Dion and Deva Premal have recorded soul inspiring pieces of music that have added so much beauty to my life and to the lives of thousands of others. These women are moved to create and sing from the very essence of their souls and that is exactly how we touch each other and make a difference in the outcome of a single life. You can change the moves any way you like, too. If any are too strenuous for you, replace them with moves that suit your physical capabilities or vice versa.

World Mantra Exercise

First, choose a space that inspires you. Then choose a song that inspires you. It is our tradition at Grail Springs to play "Aad Guray (I Bow to the Primal Wisdom)" by Deva Premal, one of the most moving and soul inspiring compositions I have ever heard. This mantra comes from the Sacred Writings of the Sanskrit.

Write out these four words on separate pieces of paper, and place each of them on the corresponding wall in the following directions: Gratitude in the East, Humility in the North, Grace in the West, and Reverence in the South. I've chosen these four words as I feel they are the most powerful in combination, however, feel free to create your own invocations using words that have meaning to you. Deva Premal's musical track is approximately six minutes long, so each segment lasts about a minute-and-a-half in each direction.

1. Facing east, start by standing straight, legs together, and arms by your side. Breathe deeply throughout this entire practice in a relaxed state, using long, smooth breaths. Now spread your feet until they are shoulder-width apart, knees slightly bent, and then stretch and raise your arms out and up to the heavens and hold them there while you breathe.

2. Bring arms down in front of you at shoulder height, while moving into a squat (knees bent, weight back on heels, toes up). Bow your head and join hands together stretched out in front of bowed head. Breathe deeply and slowly straighten up.

3. Repeat numbers 1 and 2 two more times.

4. Now standing tall, move into a balancing pose. I like to do the yoga "tree pose" here. Then follow this by moving slowly onto your other leg, hold, and then stand tall again.

5. Complete this routine by bringing hands together in Namaste, or prayer pose. Bow and let your thoughts go. Then turn to your left and begin again. Repeat this routine facing once in each direction, starting with east and finishing with a bow to the south.

Each time you face a new direction, attempt to embody the essence of the corresponding word. Fill your heart and mind with the wholeness of its meaning; first gratitude, then humility, then grace, and ending with reverence. When facing the word gratitude for instance, feel gratitude. Close your eyes and thoughtfully allow images to come to mind about everyone and everything that you feel grateful for in your life. Invite the feelings that relate to each word to wash over you, around you, and through you. The experience has been described by many people at Grail Springs as both moving and uplifting. Choosing the right piece of music that truly inspires you is very important, as the frequency of music, notes, and sounds to correspond certain frequencies of the chakra system. And the louder the better I say! Fill the room up!

The 7 Grail Essentials for a Brilliant & Vibrant Life

When you make a conscious decision to begin a new path in life, transformation has already begun. Success begins when you make small changes in your perception like when you just know it is time to give something up that is harmful to you, or add something to your life that you know could benefit you. If you've never had a rude awakening to a change in perception, then more than likely it's been a very gradual dawning. People require time to adjust to change and so do the micro rhythms or patterns within your body which have an influence on the way you feel and think. Even if you begin with small steps regarding what you eat and what you avoid, it can make a big difference in your health. Use your overall state of health and lessening of your problems in various areas as a barometer for what works for you as an individual. (e.g. Some people find that it's dairy that causes congestion, others realize after being on a detox program that it's wheat or some other food that reacts badly with their system.)

Cells have memories of their own and the neuro-network of the brain is wired in a way that has been influenced as a result of your past and present environment, your life, your habits and lifestyle choices. Those memories and patterns will change over time with new realizations and with repetition of new patterns. Pay attention to the following statement because there is no way around its truth: "Inner transformation comes by making small realizations, implementing a plan and repeating the actions – over, and over, and over again!" It takes time for new neuro pathways to be built.

Transformation occurs over time – these changes have an impact on the cellular level and in the neurons of the brain as it re-wires and re-fires. This will manifest outwardly in a recognizable change. Old habits die, and new habits are born. We have changed our perception.

Good health is not something you magically end up with. It's a constant journey, not an instant destination. The objective is to repair damage, regain the body's full strength and then maintain it at the highest level possible. Success is having patience enough to let time take its course, let the body heal, and then be committed to nurturing your continued achievements.

At Grail Springs we work with seven primary tenets in the natural health arena to achieve inner and outer transformation. You can design a solid plan incorporating each of the seven to keep that internal balance and to build and maintain optimum health for the rest of your life:

- Assessment
- A regular detox body cleanse to begin the alkalizing process
- Proper nutrition based on an acid/alkaline pH balance approach
- Fitness and movement
- Breath work and oxygen therapy to revitalize cells and tissues
- Right thought, mindfulness and meditation
- Support

 We guess, we experiment, we understand, and finally we actualize.

In this book, you will find tips and antidotes, recipes and techniques for detoxifying body, heart, and mind, and ways to reconnect with your soul. There are several methods in each of the sections that you can choose from and customize to fit your own life plan. Even for the busy person with a hectic lifestyle there will be many suggestions and techniques that you can easily do when you are traveling or have time restrictions.

First thing I suggest is to find yourself a journal. Invest in a beautiful one, something to treasure. You want to enjoy holding it, opening it, and writing in it. After all, this is your story, your grail journey. Let this be a testament to your quest for change and transformation. Someone else may benefit from your writings in the future. And that is the point. As we create change in our life, we can have a great influence on those around us and a desire to pass on what we know so that they may benefit too. Enjoy the journey!

chapter 4
Get Thee A Master Plan!

A Brilliant, Healthy Life Starts with Detox, Detox, and More Detox!

The Acid/Alkaline Phenomenon

Seasonal Detox Cleanse

3- to 7-Day Detox Cleanse

7-Day Juice Fasting Plan

Recipes from the Grail Springs Kitchen

A Brilliant Healthy Life Starts with Detox, Detox and more Detox!

"Giving the body the vacation it needs from the onslaught of chemicals and substances we ingest both voluntarily and not, on a day-to-day basis, allows healing and rebalance to begin in our body. In my practise, I usually look at the SNACC habits of sugar, nicotine, caffeine, alcohol and chemical intake and begin there with my prescription for clearing congestive and acidic symptoms as well as improving health"

– Elson M. Haas MD,
Integrated Medicine Practitioner for 35 years

Being at the top of our game is incredibly rewarding. We are rolling along, aligning ourselves with our vision, working hard to make it happen, money is abundant, our clients and staff are happy, referrals are pouring in. But all too often we are so focused on our career that we sacrifice other aspects of our life, namely our health. Everything is going great until one day the call comes in from the doctor's office, "we would like you to come in for a re-test. We just want to make sure it's nothing." We've either received a scary call like this ourselves or we know someone who has.

An increasing number of individuals are recognizing that being self-responsible for their own health and wellbeing, while focusing on disease prevention are key components to ensuring longevity. Choosing a life in balance is simply an intelligent approach to ensuring a happy, healthy, fulfilling life. Action steps towards disease prevention should start with a plan that includes a holistic detox body cleanse at the beginning of each season and a follow through using the acid/alkaline approach to diet for the rest of your life. Though there are no organized studies today on the effects of detox cleansing on long term health benefits, Grail Springs continues to be witness to the undeniable and visible effects of a holistic detox cleanse within an average stay of five to seven days.

Adopt a regular detox cleanse at the start of each season and the acid/alkaline approach to diet for the rest of your life. It's your best insurance for disease prevention and maintaining good health.

One thing that astonished us when we launched the detox program in 2004, was how quickly the body responds to the detox process. Individuals who have suffered chronic inflammation and joint pain find relief within days. Just recently we observed a woman in her sixties who could not walk without her cane when she arrived, but no longer needed it after a twelve day stay.

A detox regimen has an effect on your physical, emotional, and mental state. A greater sense of serenity, peace and calm arrives towards the latter part of a cleanse. Most people gain a more youthful appearance and a healthy, vibrant glow. The Grail Springs Detox plan is simply the best holistic, non-invasive anti-aging regimen we have seen. It is recommended that you consult with your health care provider before beginning a cleanse if you have any chronic health issues.

The Acid/Alkaline Phenomenon

Grail Springs prescribes the acid/alkaline pH balance approach to diet. I believe it saved me from a certain premature death. It sounds dramatic but it is true. This simple yet revolutionary food philosophy nourishes us by maintaining a proper pH balance in our body.

Food is probably the one area where most people will have to make the biggest change and perhaps have the most resistance. We get that. And seeing the list of the more potentially toxic and acidic foods will hardly surprise you: red meat, fast food, soda pop, refined sugar, baked goods, hydrogenated fats, and coffee, to name a few. Considered highly acidic, all of these foods create a pH imbalance and cause congestion in the colon, the leading cause of disease. Ailments often begin with constipation and other bowel problems, or with congested sinuses and continually getting sick with "colds." Continued imbalance of the acid-alkaline state can lead to health problems from inflammation, chronic fatigue, ulcers, back pain – the list goes on.

Here's a little scenario I like to share in my lectures that seems to hit home as it did with me: Remember biology 101 class? Remember the petri dish experiment with an acid gel or alkaline gel lining the bottom of the dish? The teacher would place two pieces of bacteria from the same source into the dishes, close the lids and store them in a cupboard. Left for a week or so, the acid dish would produce a disgusting green mold while the alkaline dish was clean as a whistle. Now, apply this same scenario to your body, and particularly, if you can imagine, to your colon. Your colon is dark, moist, and warm. If your colon is also sitting in a constant acidic state…well, you get the picture.

Your body is happiest in a slightly alkaline pH balanced state above 7.0 (0.0 being most acidic and 14.0 being most alkaline). The blood pH stays at about 7.41 and your body does all kinds of balancing to keep it that way. Then when we eat an acid diet, the body buffers those acids and stores them in your tissues. Acids stored in the body over a long period of time show up as congestion, swelling, inflammation and then stiffness and tissue

The acid/alkaline pH balance approach to diet is the single most important piece of information to ensure physical health and longevity!

Bacteria and disease love an acidic environment but can not flourish in an alkaline environment.

degeneration. This leads to other problems such as itchy skin, allergies, joint pain and more.

It's not that acid forming foods are bad, they just have to be balanced out with alkalizing foods when it comes to our food consumption. We do need both because of the nutrients such as minerals they each provide. There are several interpretations and acid/alkaline food charts out on the market and published in various books. Yet the rule of thumb that most agree on is to eat primarily alkaline foods for good health — that's 70–80% alkaline foods to 20–30% acidic foods.

The North American diet is the reverse of that. Most North Americans are eating closer to 80% acidic foods and only 20% alkaline foods.

The balanced alkaline diet is the missing link to achieving the appropriate weight, to achieving optimum health, and to ultimately preventing premature aging and disease. There are cookbooks now on the market that offer delicious recipes on cooking for an alkaline balanced diet. We have supplied you with over 70 delicious balanced recipes from the Grail Springs kitchen at the end of this chapter.

[
"Achieving perfect balance
depends predominantly on
understanding and applying the
acid/alkaline balance to your diet."
– Raw food guru David Wolfe
]

With steady focus, and a willingness to experiment with alternatives, acidic foods can be given up or in the very least cut back. Our chefs at Grail Springs for instance, do not use red meat, white sugar, white table salt, white flour, white rice, or wheat and use very little dairy (occasionally goat cheese).

Here are some simple replacements that you can experiment with at home:

Sugar
Replace white sugar in your house with maple syrup or agave nectar
Bonus – they are alkalizing!

Salt
Replace white salt with pink Himalayan salt
Bonus – contains no toxins and has eighty-four elements found in your body

Flour
Replace white flour with rice or spelt flour
Bonus – superior fibre resource

Rice
Replace white rice with brown rice
Bonus – higher fibre and excellent source of trace minerals which helps produce energy

Dairy
Replace cow's milk with brown rice milk, oat milk, almond milk, or hemp milk
Bonus – lactose- and cholesterol-free, and the hemp milk has omega fatty acids

> [
> "The average Western diet is tipped far
> too heavily in favour of acid foods that contain
> chemicals which give rise to a lot of miserable
> conditions such as inflammation of the joints,
> dermatitis, muscle tensions and spasms. Balancing
> this acid is the first step towards ameliorating
> these problems and feeling much healthier."
>]
> – Dr. Joshi, Author of *Holistic Detox*

It is also very important to keep your body properly mineralized. Did you know that the majority of your body's activities are powered by minerals, not vitamins? Cells contain thousands of enzymes which are only activated by minerals. Magnesium and zinc are two crucial minerals which are often deficient unless the diet consists of primarily wholesome foods. Vitamins are also important for cell function and as catalysts to biochemical reactions. B vitamins are crucial but minerals are vital Coincidentally, many minerals are found in the most alkaline of foods such as all green leafy plants like kale or spinach. Other methods of acquiring minerals into your system are via supplements and spa therapies. The spa culture, though ancient, is quite a new phenomenon in North America. Our guests are quickly realizing that some essential therapies, like our own exclusive Grail Springs Mineral Wrap, Austrian moor mud or seaweed treatments, do an excellent job removing toxins while at the same time supplying the body with minerals.

Nutrition Plan
- **Think Alkaline!** Eat a balanced alkaline/acid diet. 70 to 80 % alkaline, 20 to 30% acidic (see food list on page 65).
- **Adopt a 3- or 7-Day Detox Regimen at the beginning of each season** or as you transition into a new season. Season

changes are the stress points in our year, and we can be proactive and prevent ourselves getting sick when we give our body extra care and cleaning around these times.

- **Supplement your diet** Enlist a reputable naturally-oriented practitioner/doctor in your area. They will test your body for deficiencies and prescribe what's best for you. Your supplements could change throughout the seasons and will also change as you progressively get your body into shape and to a healthier alkaline state. And add hemp seeds to your salads everyday – they constitute one of the best mineral supplements you can take. Canada is the primary grower of this important and nutritious plant.
- **Cut out the "5 toxic whites":** white sugar, white flour, white rice, white table salt, and dairy products.
- **Eliminate red meat and soda pop altogether**
- **Purchase organic foods** whenever and wherever possible. You'll be making a contribution and doing your part to preserve and protect the planet as well as your body. Once you start on the all-organic path, you won't look back.
- **Cut your coffee intake to one cup a day, or better yet, replace your morning coffee with green tea.** Green tea can give you the caffeine boost you like to enjoy in the morning, plus you will be amazed at how different your facial skin will appear even after just a few days.
- **Add blueberries** to your grocery list every week. Add them to your meals wherever you can. Leave a bowl of them on your desk and munch on them throughout the day. They are a fantastic anti-oxidant! During the colder months, you can buy frozen organic blueberries and use them in smoothies or in other dishes.
- **Take a weekly detox bath** with seaweed, Himalayan salt crystals or moor mud from Austria. This little luxury will also supply your body with some of the necessary minerals it needs.

Proper food selection and lifestyle choices should become part of an intuitive radar process. You should get to a point when you can pick up a piece of food in a store and ask yourself, "Will this serve me or will it harm me? Is this a low energy substance or a high energy substance?"

Seasonal Detox Cleanse

A regular 3- to 7-day detox cleanse at the beginning of each season can be a practical approach even for the busiest individual. It is a safe, healthy way to kick-start the body while still being able to work and be at optimum productivity. The objective is to bring relief to the colon and gastrointestinal tract, give your body a rest and allow your inner systems to rejuvenate. A cleanse usually consists of a change in diet which means a reduction in those foods that may be regarded as acidic and congesting such as red meat, fried food, white sugar, white flour (baked goods), dairy, wheat, alcohol, and caffeine. Replace acidic food with foods that are regarded as high in alkaline and easy to digest such as vegetables, fruits, whole grains, seeds, legumes, and raw foods. Juice fasting is another popular option for detoxifying the body which we will expand on in a later chapter.

While attempting to cleanse the body it is recommended that you switch to decaf herbal tea for a week, or hot water and lemon, as an excellent alternative to coffee and one of the quickest ways to alkalize your body. Practice deep breathing, taking lots of walks outdoors, and indulge in gentle stretching, yoga or Pilates. Go easy on the cardio. Enjoying a steam room is beneficial if you have access to a fitness club, and always try to get some extra sleep. An average weight loss of a pound a day is common on a detox

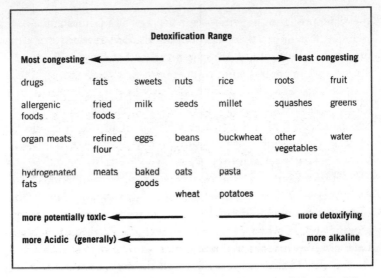

Detoxification Range

Most congesting ◀━━━━━━━━━   ━━━━━━━━━▶ least congesting

drugs	fats	sweets	nuts	rice	roots	fruit
allergenic foods	fried foods	milk	seeds	millet	squashes	greens
organ meats	refined flour	eggs	beans	buckwheat	other vegetables	water
hydrogenated fats	meats	baked goods	oats	pasta		
			wheat	potatoes		

more potentially toxic ◀━━━━━━━   ━━━━━━━▶ more detoxifying

more Acidic (generally) ◀━━━━━━   ━━━━━━▶ more alkaline

From *The New Detox Diet*, Elson M. Haas, M.D., with Daniella Chace, M.S., C.N
(Ten Speed Press, Berkeley/Toronto: 2004)

cleanse, a little more for men, with a predominantly noticeable increase in vital energy and mental clarity towards the middle to end of the week.

Dr. Elson Haas, a.k.a. "America's Detox Doc" and Integrated Medicine Physician, a good friend and advisor to Grail Springs, says detox cleansing is the missing link in modern day nutrition and is valuable for boosting the inner systems, weight loss, and overall health and well-being. This is exactly what we are witnessing at Grail Springs. We are fortunate to be able to assist individuals for an average of one week stays and observe their process from beginning to end. When it comes to weight loss, I am convinced without a doubt that when you give the body a chance to function normally, it automatically regulates closer to a person's ideal weight. For instance, a couple will check in, the man weighing in fifty pounds over his ideal weight and the woman only a few pounds over hers. Though they are both on the same program, he will lose an average of a pound and a half per day totalling ten to eleven pounds with no adverse side effects. On the contrary. And she on the other hand will experience a two or three pound total weight loss, arrive at her ideal weight and stay there. Both will have lost inches, toned up, gained a healthy glow, rid themselves of inflammation, bloating, and pain, and regained a greater sense of vitality. With hundreds of visitors entering the program each year, we see this exact same scenario over and over again.

Mental preparation is necessary; however, most individuals are so impressed with the immediate results that they become committed to an ongoing detox plan. It is never recommended to do a detox cleanse when you are ill or pregnant. Wait until you are feeling somewhat balanced and then begin.

You should expect the body to go through a natural process that will take you on a bit of an emotional and mental ride depending how far to the left on the illness-wellness continuum you have gone. My recommendation is to adopt a simple mantra which is what I do when I am on a detox program, "Go with the flow!" and it will be easier to navigate through it. The first time is always the most challenging. But once you feel the rewards, you will look forward to the second one. And before you know it, you will be so inspired by the results that you will embrace it each season with open arms for the rest of your life.

Within the first two days, expect to go through what I call a decompression period. You may feel quite lethargic, headachy and even irritable, especially if you are a heavy consumer of caffeine or sugar. Sleep when and if you can. There are a few people

The key to weight management is detox cleansing, not counting calories.

who feel restless but most want to sleep quite a bit. I call the third and fourth day the "neutral zone." That's when you feel neither good nor bad. You are just kind of floating, nothing too exciting is happening yet, but you may begin to sense what it might be like to feel pain-free and most people comment on how foreign that feels at first. We get so used to carrying on through our stress and pain we adapt to it and think of it as normal.

The pay off to your commitment starts to be seen and felt by the fifth, six and most certainly by the seventh day. That is when strength returns. We feel undeniably energized. Skin starts to glow and even the whites of our eyes get brighter. Detox cleansing represents the next wave in health and healing, a must for everybody who wants to ensure a life in balance.

Why someone might choose to go on a detox program:

- You rely on coffee, nicotine, sugar, or other junk food to keep you going
- You live in an inner-city environment and are subject to pollution and chlorinated water
- You recently stopped taking prescription drugs or pain killers
- You generally feel tired, can't sleep, and are sluggish or congested
- You suffer from constant bloating, poor digestion, gas, or constipation
- You feel or see a quickening of aging symptoms
- You are under a great deal of stress

Individuals with the following symptoms can benefit from this program:

- Headaches and migraines
- Joint pain or stiffness, chronic tension between shoulder blades
- Unhealthy skin, itchy skin

- Constipation, poor digestion, water retention, bloating
- Low energy, mental sluggishness or fogginess
- Anxiety, depression, premenstrual symptoms
- Excess dietary protein, problems losing weight
- Use of antibiotics, tetracycline, or medications for pain
- Bad breath, foot odour, or excessive sweating
- Allergies, chronic sinus congestion
- Chemical sensitivity, exposure to pollution, solvents, or other chemicals
- Consumption of alcohol, caffeine, fast food, processed food
- Emotional stress and anxiety

Precaution: If you are experiencing any of the following conditions, you should seek the advice of a physician first: chronic illness, diabetes, low blood sugar, eating disorders, thyroid disorders (high or low function), and cancer. Pregnant or lactating women should not detox.

Tips for Preparation prior to a Detox Cleanse:
- Enrol the support of a recommended naturopathic or naturally-oriented doctor and follow his or her direction to enhance the experience.
- Enrol the support of your in-house family members. If you can, encourage all the adult members to join you in your detox.
- Pick a specific date, perhaps Sunday to Sunday, and begin to prepare yourself mentally a few weeks before.
- On the Saturday prior to your start day, make sure your grocery list is in order and you have a pretty good idea as to how the week is going to unfold.
- If possible, try to fit your detox regimen into to the new moon phase for optimum detoxification results.
- Begin to cut back on red meat, white sugar, and soda pop five to seven days prior.

- Gradually reduce your caffeine intake five days prior to avoid headaches.
- Reduce your work load in preparation to take it a bit easier the week of your detox.
- If you are a smoker who is looking to quit, begin to slowly reduce the number of cigarettes per day (note that this detox program is not a smoking cessation program although people try it as a first step approach). When we alkalize the body, the cravings for nicotine and other substances lessen.
- Do not eat after 7:00 PM.
- Start going to bed a little earlier and rising earlier – 10:00 PM to 6:00 AM is ideal.

3- to 7-Day Detox Cleanse
Check List
Once you are ready to go into full swing these are some general food guidelines for you to follow for a gentle first level detox cleanse with solid food:

Eliminate:
- White sugar
- Soda pop
- Red meat
- White flour products
- Gluten, wheat and yeast products
- Soy products with the exception of miso
- White vinegar
- Caffeine
- Alcohol
- Recreational drugs
- Dairy products (with the exception of non-fat yogurt in moderation)
- White table salt (replace with Himalayan salt)
- Artificial or processed foods

**Add to your diet the following
(organic wherever available):**

- Drink lots of hot water with lemons
  (not to replace regular water)
- Drink lots of plain water (about 1 litre, but no more
  than 4 ounces while eating)
- Decaffeinated herbal teas
- Wheatgrass and fresh sprouts if you have access
- Homemade vegetable juices if possible
- Brown rice, oatmeal
- Dressings made with olive oil (good fat) and lemon
- Hemp milk, rice milk, and almond milk
- Egg yolk but only a couple of times in the week
- Miso and non-fat yogurt (in moderation)
- Gluten-free, wheat-free products
- Fish (exclude shellfish)
- Poultry (moderate)

7-Day Juice Fasting Plan

Once you have experienced an introductory detox plan with
solid food you might consider your next detox experience to be
a juice fasting plan. Again, it takes mental preparation prior to
starting a juice fasting plan but it is one of the fastest ways to
restore your health. You will undoubtedly experience the significant healing power of fresh juice to feel young and look great.
Most people get hooked once they've tried it successfully even
just once.

When one thinks of juice fasting, most people think of fruit
juices. Regular juice fasters typically eliminate fruit juice juices
altogether. That choice is yours and should be guided by your
blood sugar levels and your own knowledge of your health condition. It is important to listen to your body. First time juicers
will often find they have to add some extra protein powder in
their morning beverage. Nut milks like hemp and almond are

also good alternatives for adding a bit of protein to your diet if needed. Hot vegetable broths are an alternative to your evening beverage.

Spring and autumn are the best times to do a juice fast. If you are choosing to do one in the winter, adjust your plan to include some protein in the morning and include warm broths at night. If you are in a region where the winters are very cold with extreme temperatures choose to do a first level detox instead with solid food rather than a full juice fast. See the recipe section for dishes to prepare for a first level detox.

Benefits of a juice fasting cleanse program:
- Rid your body of damaging toxins
- Heal chronic ailments without drugs
- Give cells an opportunity to cleanse, heal and rejuvenate
- Find levels of energy you only dream of
- Lose a healthy amount of weight, fast
- Lower cholesterol levels
- Clean and replenish your colon
- Bring clarity to mind and spirit

Who might be ready for a juice fasting cleanse?
The predominant motivation for going on a juice fast is for physical healing or renewal. More and more individuals are choosing to integrate this ancient practice as a regular health maintenance and detoxification regimen into their life. Many people practice it for disease prevention and sometimes even for treatment of disease. Either way, successful juice fasting comes from an inner desire when a person is mentally motivated and prepared. Juice fasting can increase energy and extend life. Another major reason why people choose to fast is for weight loss or to relieve themselves of food addictions, substance addictions and other habits that take their toll on the body. With busy

lifestyles this becomes an excellent solution for those living a hectic life with time restraints.

General guidelines to follow for a juice fasting cleanse:

- Drink 10 to 12 ounces of fresh homemade juices every two hours from 8:00 AM to 6:00 PM (see recipe section for ideas).
- Drink 2 litres of hot water with lemons throughout the day (not to replace regular water).
- Drink at least 1 litre of filtered water throughout the day especially when you feel hungry.
- You may use the Master Cleanse recipe (see page 77) several times during the day and in-between your juicing hours
- Decaffeinated herbal teas are acceptable throughout your day until 8:00 PM
- A 2-ounce shot of wheatgrass (see page 69), apple cider vinegar or a teaspoon of Austrian moor mud stirred in a glass of water and taken first thing in the morning on an empty stomach is a great start to your day. It dissolves the acid levels and raises your alkaline levels among many other benefits.

Wheatgrass is considered the King of Juice. It purifies and alkalizes the blood, neutralizes toxins, cleanses the liver and colon, oxygenates the cells, and detoxifies the cellular fluids. It's high in chlorophyll, which is a natural detoxifier. Wheatgrass requires a specific wheatgrass juicer. You can also buy it in flash-frozen form at your local whole foods suppliers.

All of the following fruits, vegetables, and spices have great health benefits and can be used in combination. Carrot, cucumber and apple make a good base for any added combinations (see page 80 for recipe ideas).

- wheatgrass, spinach, kale, carrot, tomato, cabbage,
  beet, cucumber, lemon, parsley, alfalfa sprouts,
  ginger, and seasonings such as dill, garlic and cayenne
- Best fruits: apple, papaya, mango, watermelon,
  pineapple
- Best toxins absorbing foods: beet, watermelon,
  apple, and red grape juice

The following is an excellent general guideline that we follow at Grail Springs. It suits most individuals who are starting out. Once you have completed a couple of juice fasting regimens, you can decide how you want to change it up to suit your body and your needs:

6:00 AM	2 ounces of straight wheat grass or
	2 ounces apple cider vinegar or
	1 teaspoon of Austrian moor mud stirred into
	6 ounces of water; wait 10 minutes then enjoy
	some decaffeinated herbal tea
8:00 AM	12 ounces fruit juice (with protein powder
	if needed)
10:00 AM	12 ounces fruit juice mixed with
	vegetable juice
12:00 PM	12 ounces vegetable juice
2:00 PM	12 ounces vegetable juice
4:00 PM	12 ounces vegetable juice
6:00 PM	12 ounces vegetable juice or hot broth
8:00 PM	decaffeinated herbal tea or water
	(optional)

Recommended Juicing Machine

Most health care practitioners who promote juice fasting cleanses recommend the Omega Juicer series. When purchasing your own machine, which can be a hefty investment, be sure you are considering quality, performance, and price. Not all juicers are built or function the same. There is quite a variety out there.

Compare before you shop. From our experience, most juicers can only be purchased online so anticipate a few weeks for delivery. Note: a regular juicer and a wheatgrass juicer are two completely different juicers.

After a Juice Fasting Cleanse

A juice fasting cleanse can be a remarkable experience with remarkable results. Transitioning back to a regular diet is tricky but can be made simple. For the couple of days coming off your juice fast, integrate the following:

- Start each morning by drinking warm water with lemon.
- Enjoy fruit smoothies for breakfast made with almond, hemp, or rice milk.
- Add protein powders to your breakfast drink.
- Prepare steamed vegetables for lunch and dinner with a bit of brown rice.
- Hot broths are wonderful with a few vegetables.
- Enjoy light salads with an olive oil dressing.

After the second day you can introduce the following, keeping in mind that you really want to stay on a vegetarian diet for the rest of the week:

- Hot quinoa for breakfast or steel cut oats
- Other cooked whole grains such as rice or millet
- Limited whole grain bread
- Sprouts, seeds, and legumes
- Soups
- Fruits and vegetables

The best advice of all is to subscribe to the acid/alkaline approach to diet for the rest of your life!

Recipes

Detoxifying Cocktails and Juice Fasting Recipes ..
Grail Springs Detoxifying Elixir • Dr. Haas' Detoxifying Cinnamon
Elixir • Autumn Rejuvenation Ration • The Master Cleanse •
Morning Calm • Eye Opener • Morning Mantra • Mineral Tonic •
Immune Builder • Tomato Talk • Green Machine

Smoothies & Shakes....
Hawaiian Medley • Cool Breeze • Papaya Moonlight • Mango
Madness • Sunflower-Banana Shake

Breakfast....
Millet with Mandarin Orange • Grail's Great Granola • Lemon
Scented Poached Eggs • Maple Syrup Crepes • Blueberry and
Ginger Pancakes • Hemp and Spinach Frittatas • Morning Health
Muffins • Tropical Sunrise Mousse • Ginger Date Dessert for
Breakfast

Soups, Salads, and Lunch Fare......
Shitake Ginger Soup • Spinach Lemon Soup • Carrot and Orange
Soup • Chilled Lemony Pea Soup • Ginger Miso Soup • Roasted
Garlic Soup • Parsnip Soup • Parsnip & Apple Bisque • Power of
Beets Borscht • Butternut Squash & Fennel Soup • Marinated Tofu
Salad • Asparagus and Salmon Salad • Basil, Orange, and Peach
Salad • Broccoli, Tomato, and Watercress Salad • Arame Salad •
Crispy Sesame Tofu • Watermelon and Mango Salad with Citrus
Dressing • Southwestern Caesar Salad • Warm Chickpea Salad •
Mediterranean Quinoa Salad • Sacred Millet Salad • Dolmas with
Goat Cheese and Cranberries • Beet in a Blanket

Mains...

California Girl Roasted Root Veggie Sushi • Chickpea Croquettes • Sweet Yellow Pepper Gazpacho • Ginger "Veggie Beef" & Buckwheat • Chilly Day Chili • Quinoa & Kale Stuffed Tomatoes • Quinoa & Kale Stuffed Tomatoes • Salmon en Papillote • Orange Roughy with Ginger Sesame Marinade • Salsa Borracha on Red Snapper • Poached Lemongrass Red Snapper with Quinoa • Miso Marinated Salmon • Ginger and Green Onion Tilapia • Pecan Crusted Chicken with Mustard Sauce • Cucumber and Feta Salsa with Grilled Chicken • South American Vegetable Stew

Sides, Sauces, and Snacks....

Braised Fennel with Orange and Walnuts • Red Rice Stuffing • Dijon Sweet Potatoes • Braised Radishes and Apples • Healthy Cheeseless Cheese Dip • Flax Tomato Crackers • Yogurt Cheese • Red Lentil Dahl • Gomashio • Arugula Pesto • Cilantro Pesto • Lime Scented Spinach Spread • Sprouted Garbanzo Hummus • Nutmeg Sauce • Braised Artichokes and Peas • Spring Rolls with Spicy Almond Sauce • Quinoa Fennnel Pilaf • Cashew Cream Sauce • Tahini-Garlic Sauce • Dancing Beans Salsa • Mango Chutney • Asparagus Spears & Cashew "Cream" • Sunflower Seed Pate • Raw Nut "Cream" • "Angry-Style" Ancient Grain

Desserts...

Dr. Haas' Banana Nice Cream • Chocolate Torte • Cocunut Cream Pie • Gingerbread • Bean Brownie • Spiced Cashew Ice Cream • Raw Carrot Cake • Truffles for Angels

Detoxifying Cocktails

These are great health tonics that encourage detoxification, raise alkalinity and build the immune system.

Grail Springs Detox Elixir

This refreshing detox cocktail is a favourite at Grail Springs, served daily to guests on our health and wellness programs, as well as at our traveling Detox Beverage Bar, which is invited to many celebrity and fundraising functions. The Grail Springs Detox Elixir reduces acidity and raises the alkaline levels of the body. Though lemons are thought of as highly acidic, when they mix with digestive juices and get utilized in the body, they become more alkaline. Maple syrup is also surprisingly alkalizing for the body, an excellent substitute for white sugar in any cooking. Ginger is a fantastic digestive cure and immune supporter. We recommend using all organic products. In the summer months, Perrier is a great choice for the added bubbly because it contains no additives. You can make the infusion ahead of time and store it for days in the refrigerator. This is a wonderful and refreshing and healthy drink that the whole family with love. Excellent served with hot water in the winter too.

Juice from 2 to 3 organic lemons

1/4 cup (50 ml) finely chopped organic ginger

1/3 cup (75 ml) organic maple syrup (or to taste)

- Infuse the above three ingredients for at least 30 minutes
- Just before serving add 2 tablespoons (30 ml) of mixture to glass.
- Top with ice cold Perrier or hot water.
- Stir well.
- Garnish with blueberry and mint leaf if you wish.

Serves 2–3

Dr. Haas' Detoxifying Cinnamon Cider

2 cups (500 ml) organic unsweetened apple cider
   or apple juice
1/4 teaspoon (1 ml) ground cinnamon
1/4 teaspoon (1 ml) ground ginger
2 teaspoons (10 ml) pure maple syrup
1/2 an orange, sliced
1/4 teaspoon (1 ml) ground cardamom
Fresh, peeled ginger slices

- In a saucepan heat the apple cider over low heat.
- Add cinnamon, ginger, maple syrup, and any other spices desired to the cider.
- Place orange slices in mug and add cardamom and fresh ginger.
- Pour hot cider into mugs and serve hot.

Serves 2

Autumn Rejuvenation Ration

3 cups (750 ml) spring water

1 tablespoon (15 ml) chopped ginger root

1–2 tablespoons (15–30 ml) miso paste

1–2 stalks green onion, chopped

Chopped cilantro, to taste

1–2 pinches cayenne pepper

2 teaspoons (10 ml) extra virgin olive oil

Juice of 1/2 lemon

Boil water. Add ginger root. Simmer 10 minutes. Stir in miso paste to taste (do not allow miso paste to boil). Turn off burner. Then add green onion, cilantro, cayenne, olive oil, and lemon juice. Remove from stove and cover to steep for 10 minutes. You may vary ingredient portions to satisfy your palate. Enjoy.

From *The New Detox Diet*, Elson M. Haas, M.D., with Daniella Chace, M.S., C.N
(Ten Speed Press, Berkeley/Toronto: 2004)

The Master Cleanse

This is a 50-year-old diet that was invented by Stanley Burroughs. This version comes from Dr. Haas' book *The New Detox Diet*. Many people swear by this diet and will drink only the Master Cleanse for several days. We like it served warm or even hot at Grail Springs.

    2 tablespoons (30 ml) freshly squeezed lemon or
        lime juice
    1 tablespoon (15 ml) pure maple syrup
        (up to 2 tablespoons if you want to drop less weight)
    1/10 teaspoon (0.5 ml) cayenne pepper
    1 cup (250 ml) spring water

Important Notes: Mix and drink 8–12 glasses throughout the day. Eat and drink nothing else except water, laxative herb tea, and peppermint chamomile tea. Keep the mixture in a glass container (not plastic) or make it fresh each time. Rinse you mouth with water after each glass to prevent the lemon juice from hurting the enamel of your teeth.

From *The New Detox Diet*, Elson M. Haas, M.D., with Daniella Chace, M.S., C.N
(Ten Speed Press, Berkeley/Toronto: 2004)

Some Benefits of Fasting

Purification

Rejuvenation

More energy

Rest for digestive organs

Greater abdominal peace

Clearer skin

Sense of personal beauty

Anti-aging effects

Improved senses: vision, hearing, taste

Self-confidence

Reduction of allergies

Weight loss

Clothes fit more comfortably

Drug detoxification

Better resistance to disease

Spiritual awareness

More restful sleep

More relaxation

Greater motivation and optimism

New inspiration and creativity

More clarity, mental and emotional

Improved communications

Better organization

Cleaner boundaries for energy in and out

Commitment to habit changes

Diet changes, long term

Contradictions for Fasting

Underweight

Fatigue

Low immunity

Weak heart

Low blood pressure

Cardiac arrhythmias

Cold weather

Pregnancy

Nursing

Pre- and post-surgery

Cancer

Peptic ulcers

Nutritional deficiencies

Children

From *The New Detox Diet*, Elson M. Haas, M.D., with Daniella Chace, M.S., C.N
(Ten Speed Press, Berkeley/Toronto: 2004)

Juice Fasting Recipes

There are no rules to creating your own juice fasting recipes. However, if you are going to add fruit to your juice fasting day, make sure that your fruit intake happens in the morning hours only. Fruit juices are great energy builders and high in calories. Ease off towards the early afternoon. Experiment and add your own ingredients.

Whenever possible, use all organic fresh fruit and vegetables.

Note: In the following recipes you may add garlic to taste.

Garlic has been found to:
- lower blood sugar levels in diabetics
- promote detoxification reactions
- boost the immune system
- protect against cancer
- be an antifungal

Morning Calm

2 cucumbers
8 stalks of celery
8 kale leaves (stalk and leaf)
1/4 inch (6 mm) piece of ginger

Eye Opener

2 cucumbers
Juice of 1/2 lemon
2 garlic cloves
1/2 head cabbage
1/2 bunch of cilantro

Morning Mantra

8–10 stalks celery
1/2 bunch spinach
1/2 head cabbage
1/2 bunch of parsley
1/2 lemon
Fennel to taste
Tamari to taste

Mineral Tonic

1/2 bunch parsley
1/2 bunch cilantro
2 turnip leaves
3 kale leaves
6 carrots

Immune Builder

6 stalks celery
6 carrots
2 garlic cloves
1/4 bunch parsley
1/2 bunch cilantro

Tomato Talk

3 tomatoes
1/4 bunch spinach
1 green pepper
Handful parsley
Tamari to taste

Green Machine

1 bunch alfalfa sprouts
4 stalks celery
2 cucumbers
4 beet greens
1/4 bunch spinach
4 collard green leaves
1/4 inch (6 mm) piece of ginger
Lemon to taste

Fruit Juices and the Organs or Conditions They Help Heal

Lemon – liver, gallbladder, allergies,
    asthma, cardiovascular disease
    (CVD), colds
Citrus – CVD, obesity, hemorrhoids,
    varicose veins
Apple – liver, intestines
Pear – gallbladder
Grape – colon, anemia
Papaya – stomach, indigestion,
    hemmorhoids, colitis
Pineapple – allergies, arthritis,
    inflammation, edema, hemorrhoids
Watermelon – kidneys, edema
Black cherry – colon, menstrual
    problems, gout

Vegetable Juices and the Organs or Conditions They Help Heal

Greens – CVD, skin, eczema,
    digestive problems, obesity,
    bad breath
Spinach – anemia, eczema
Parsley – kidneys, edema, arthritis
Beet Greens – gallbladder, liver,
    osteoporosis
Watercress – anemia, colds
Wheat grass – anemia, liver, intestines,
    bad breath
Cabbage – colitis, ulcers
Carrots – eyes, arthritis, osteoporosis
Beets – blood, liver, menstrual problems,
    arthritis
Celery – kidneys, diabetes, osteoporosis
Cucumber – edema, diabetes
Jerusalem artichokes – diabetes
Garlic – allergies, colds, hypertension,
    CVD, high fats, diabetes
Radish – liver, high fats, obesity
Potatoes – intestines, ulcers

Smoothies & Shakes

All of these can be put in the blender with 1 cup or so of crushed ice and you can also add a splash or more of sparkling water to taste.

Hawaiian Medley
1/2 a pineapple
1/2 cup (125 ml) blueberries
Perrier to taste

Cool Breeze
1 medium bunch red grapes
2 cups watermelon with rind
1 orange
2 or 3 mint leaves

Papaya Moonlight
1 small papaya or 1/4 of a large papaya
1 large apple
1/4 lime

Mango Madness
1 large juicy mango
1/2 pineapple
1/2 cup (125 ml) strawberries or blueberries

Makes between 1 and 2 servings

Sunflower-Banana Shake

1 cup (250 ml) sunflower seeds, raw and soaked

2 cups (500 ml) water, as needed for consistency

2 cups (500 ml) ice, optional

1 large banana, ripe

1/2 teaspoon (5 ml) vanilla, or to taste

1 tablespoon (15 ml) maple syrup, or to taste

- Soak sunflower seeds in 8 cups (2 L) of water overnight in the refrigerator. Drain.
- Blend ingredients together, adding vanilla and maple syrup to taste.

Patty James Cooking School and Nutrition Centre for Grail Springs

Breakfast

Millet with Mandarin Oranges

Almond Milk

Soak 1 cup (250 ml) raw almonds overnight in cold water. The next morning drain water and place almonds in blender with 4 cups (1 L) of fresh water and blend until very smooth, Strain through cheesecloth, without squeezing. Refrigerate.

2/3 cup (150 ml) millet, washed

2 cups (500 ml) orange juice

1 cinnamon stick

3 pods cardamom

1 pinch of Himalayan salt

1/2 cup (125 ml) almond milk

1 Mandarin orange

1 date, chopped

Dry millet and toast it by stirring constantly in a saucepan for 3 minutes. Add orange juice, cinnamon stick, cardamom pods and salt. Bring to a boil, lower heat to a simmer, cover and let simmer for 30 minutes. Remove cardamom pods and cinnamon stick. Ladle into bowls and top with almond milk, mandarin orange slices and sprinkle with chopped date.

Serves 3

Patty James Cooking School and Nutrition Centre for Grail Springs

Grail's Great Granola

4 cups (1 L) old-fashion oats

1 1/2 cups (375 ml) sliced almonds

1/2 cup (125 ml) raw sugar

1/2 teaspoon (2.5 ml) Himalayan salt

1/2 teaspoon (2.5 ml) cinnamon

1/4 cup (50 ml) grape seed oil

1/4 cup (50 ml) honey

1 teaspoon (5 ml) pure vanilla extract

- Preheat oven to 300F.
- In a bowl mix oats, almonds, raw sugar, salt, and cinnamon.
- In a saucepan warm the oil and honey. Whisk in vanilla.
- Carefully pour the liquid over the oat mixture. Stir gently with a wooden spoon
- Finish mixing by hand. Spread granola in a 15 x10 baking sheet.
- Bake 40 minutes, stirring every 10 minutes.
- Transfer pan to a rack to cool completely.
- Seal granola in an airtight container or sealable plastic bag.
- Store at room temperature for up to 1 week or freeze up to 3 months.
- Serve with yogurt and fresh berries or fruit. Yum!

Serves 4–6

Lemon Scented Poached Eggs

2 eggs
1/4 cup (50 ml) water
2 tablespoons (30 ml) lemon juice
4 stalks asparagus
1 toasted whole grain bread slice
1 teaspoon (5 ml) butter

- Place fresh lemon juice in room temperature water and let sit for 5 minutes; strain out pulp.
- Steam asparagus for 2 minutes (or until al dente) and keep warm.
- Heat a small frying pan over medium heat; brush with olive oil. Crack in 2 eggs and pour in the lemon water very slowly, careful to pour the water next to the eggs, not on them.
- Cover and cook until desired softness – generally 2–3 minutes for a runny yolk.
- While the eggs are cooking, cut out a circle from the toasted slice of bread – you can use a cookie cutter (save the crusts for bread crumbs.) Brush with a bit of butter.
- Arrange eggs on toast and attractively place asparagus on top. Garnish with lemon peel and a sprig of parsley. Serve at once

Serves 1

Patty James Cooking School and Nutrition Centre for Grail Springs

Maple Syrup Crepes

2 cups (500 ml) almond or rice milk

1 cup (250 ml) flour

2 egg whites

1 egg

1 tablespoon (15 ml) maple syrup

1 tablespoon (15 ml) walnut oil

1/8 teaspoon (0.625 ml) Himalayan salt

- Combine all ingredients in blender or food processor; blend until smooth.
- Let sit for 30 minutes.
- Rub an 8-inch skillet with an oiled paper towel; heat over medium-high heat.
- Spoon 3–4 tablespoons crepe batter into skillet, tilting and rotating skillet to cover evenly with batter.
- Cook until edges begin to brown, about 1 1/2 minutes.
- Turn crepe over and cook until lightly browned, about 30 seconds.
- Remove crepe to plate to cool. Repeat process with remaining batter.
- Place parchment paper in-between crepes while cooling.
- Fold attractively and serve with nutmeg sauce (see page 155) and fresh berries.

Yield: 12 crepes

Patty James Cooking School and Nutrition Centre for Grail Springs

Blueberry & Ginger Pancakes

1 cup (250 ml) whole wheat organic flour

1 teaspoon (5 ml) baking powder

1 teaspoon (5 ml) baking soda

Dash of Himalayan salt

2 teaspoons (10 ml) fresh ginger, chopped

1 tablespoon (15 ml) pure maple syrup

1 cup (250 ml) almond milk or rice milk

1 tablespoon (15 ml) almond oil

1 teaspoon (5 ml) vanilla

1 egg yolk, lightly beaten

1 egg white, stiffly beaten

1 cup (250 ml) fresh blueberries

1/3 cup (75 ml) vanilla yogurt (garnish)

Pure maple syrup to taste

- Sift dry ingredients together.
- Whip egg white and set aside.
- Mix maple syrup with almond milk, ginger, oil and vanilla, then beat in the egg yolk.
- Make a well in the centre of the dry ingredients and pour in the wet ingredients, mixing only until just blended.
- Carefully fold in beaten egg white, followed by blueberries.
- Heat griddle over medium heat. Oil lightly, then immediately pour 2 tablespoons (30 ml) of batter onto griddle to form small medallions.
- Turn heat down to medium-low and continue cooking until golden brown on the bottom side and bubbly on top. Flip and cook until underside is golden brown.
- Serve with a dollop of vanilla yogurt and a drizzle of pure maple syrup.

Serves 2

Hemp & Spinach Frittatas

7 eggs

1/2 cup (125 ml) hemp milk

11/2 teaspoons (7.5 ml) chopped garlic

1/2 tsp (2.5 ml) Himalayan salt

2 teaspoons (10 ml) olive oil

1 cup (250 ml) fresh spinach leaves

1 tomato, diced

Fresh basil leaves

Fresh oregano leaves

1/3 cup (75 ml) feta cheese

- Whip eggs in bowl with hemp milk, garlic, and salt.
- Add oil to a cast iron pan on medium heat.
- Sauté spinach leaves. Once spinach has darkened, add egg mixture and tomatoes.
- Cover with lid for 4 minutes.
- Remove lid and bake in oven under broiler until egg mixture has nicely browned.
- Garnish with chopped fresh basil, oregano and a sprinkle of feta cheese.

Serves 4

Morning Health Muffins

A dozen of these super-healthy super-food bran muffins will go a long way. Grab one or two on your way out the door for a breakfast on the go that'll activate your digestive system and sweep clean your intestinal walls. They contain no eggs or dairy, no fat, no refined sugar, and are packed with power.

Endless variations are possible, depending what fruit is in season or in your freezer. Substitute raisins, gogi berries, apples, cranberries, mango pieces or peaches for blueberries.

If you prepare the ingredients the night before, when you wake up it's simply a matter of combining wet with dry, then popping them in the oven. You can go off and do your morning ritual for half an hour, then come back to fresh baked morning muffin goodness.

2 cups organic wheat bran

2 cups organic spelt flour

1 tsp baking soda

2 tsp baking powder

pinch cinnamon

half a tsp Himalayan sea salt

handful each, organic sunflower seeds, organic sesame seeds

1/2 cup of maple syrup

1 1/2 cup of unsweetened juice of any kind
    (apple, orange, cranberry, mango)

1 tsp pure vanilla extract

1 cup fresh or frozen blueberries

- Ten minute prep:
- Mix dry ingredients in a large bowl.
- In a large glass measuring cup, stir together wet ingredients.
- Add liquid to dry and mix thoroughly. Add blueberries and stir in gently.
- Drop into lightly oiled muffin tins and bake for half an hour at 350.
- When you take the muffins out of the oven, allow them to sit in the pan for a few minutes before lifting them out. Eat warm with your morning cup of chai or green tea.

Yield: 1 dozen

Tropical Sunrise Mousse

1 package firm "silken" tofu
1 1/2 ripe mango, peeled and sliced
1/2 ripe banana, peeled and sliced
1 1/2 tsp pure vanilla extract
1/4 cup pure maple syrup (or to taste)
2 tbsp fresh grated organic coconut

- Blend all ingredients except coconut in a cuisinart until smooth and creamy. Pour into champagne flutes or martini glasses and let set in fridge for 10 minutes or longer.
- Lightly toast coconut and sprinkle on top.
- This is especially good when the mangoes are ripe and in season, but variations can be made using any fruit – peach, apricot, lime, mandarin...
- Garnish with an edible flower or a gingersnap and serve.

Serves 4

Ginger Date Dessert for Breakfast

This is an extremely healthy version of the classic date square and contains too much energy for an after dinner dessert. But eaten for breakfast, or as a power boost mid-day, a little piece of this will get you movin' and groovin'.

2 cups pitted organic dates

2-inch piece of fresh ginger, minced

1 1/2 tsp pure vanilla extract

2 cups organic oats

1/2 cup organic walnuts, chopped

1 1/2 tsp cinnamon

1 tsp Himalayan sea salt

1/2 lemon

6 tbsp maple syrup

4 tbsp spring water

1 tsp coconut oil

- In a saucepan combine dates, ginger and vanilla with just enough water to cover them and bring to a boil. Turn down to minimum, and when dates begin to soften, mash them with a wooden spoon until you have a nice thick date "jam".
- In a dry frying pan on medium-high, toss oats and walnuts with cinnamon and sea salt until lightly toasted and aromatic.
- Lightly oil a small square pan with coconut oil. Dust the bottom of pan with oats and walnuts mixture.
- Pour the date mixture in, then cover with oats and walnuts.
- In a glass measuring cup, combine juice of lemon with maple syrup and spring water, then drizzle over the date squares.
- Bake at about 350 for 20 minutes.

Soups, Salads, and Lunch Fare

Shitake Ginger Soup

6 cups (1500 ml) organic vegetable or chicken stock

1 teaspoon (5 ml) fresh garlic, finely chopped

1 tablespoon (15 ml) ginger, finely chopped

1 tablespoon (15 ml) shallots, minced

1/4 cup (50 ml) fresh squeezed lemon juice

1 tablespoon (15 ml) sesame oil

4 cups (1 L) shitake mushrooms, sliced

2 tablespoons (30 ml) Bragg liquid aminos

1 tablespoon (15 ml) miso paste

1 tablespoon (15 ml) fresh chives chopped

- Sauté the garlic, ginger, shallots in sesame oil for 3 minutes on medium heat.
- Add remaining ingredients except miso and chives.
- Bring to simmer, cover, and continue to simmer for 15 minutes.
- Add miso paste just before serving.
- Garnish with fresh chives.

Serves 6

Spinach Lemon Soup

Serve Hot or Cold

   3 tablespoons (45 ml) olive oil

   1 large sweet onion, finely chopped

   1 pound (250 g) fresh spinach, washed

   3 tablespoons (45 ml) brown rice

   1 10-oz (300 g) package frozen peas

   3 tablespoons (45 m) chopped fresh dill

   4 cups (1 L) organic vegetable stock

   Himalayan salt, and nutmeg to taste

   Grated peel of 1/2 lemon

   1 cup (250 ml) yogurt plus 4 tablespoons (60ml)

   4 scallions, sliced diagonally

- Warm the oil in a large saucepan and sauté the onion until tender.
- Add the spinach and stir until it wilts. To keep the soup a bright green do not overcook or cover the spinach.
- Add the rice and peas and toss well. Stir in the dill.
- Pour in the vegetable stock and add salt, pepper and nutmeg to taste.
- Stir in the lemon peel.
- Bring to a boil, reduce the heat and simmer for 30 minutes or until the rice is tender.
- Puree the soup in a food processor. Chill for one hour.
- Before serving, stir in 1 cup of yogurt. Taste and adjust seasonings.
- To serve, place a spoonful of yogurt on each serving and scallions and a thin slice of lemon peel on top.

Serves 4

Carrot and Orange Soup

1 tablespoon (15 ml) olive oil

2 leeks, thinly sliced

6 large carrots, sliced

2 tablespoons (30 ml) curry powder

1 tablespoon (15 ml) grated lemon rind

1 cup (250 ml) organic orange juice

1 1/2 cups (375 ml) coconut milk

2 cups (500 ml) vegetable stock

1/3 cup (75 ml) organic goat milk yogurt

2/3 cup (150 ml) cashew nuts, roasted, chopped

- Heat oil in saucepan over medium heat.
- Add leeks. Sauté for 5 minutes until golden.
- Add carrots, curry powder, lemon rind, organic orange juice and stock.
- Bring to a boil. Simmer for 10 minutes.
- Cool slightly. Puree soup. Return soup to a clean saucepan. Add coconut milk.
- Heat for 4 or 5 minutes or until hot.
- Serve soup topped with yogurt, nuts and mint (optional).

Serves 4

Chilled Lemony Pea Soup

2 teaspoons (10 ml) olive oil

1/4 cup (50 ml) shallots

2 cups (500 ml) chicken or vegetable broth

2 teaspoons (10 ml) cornstarch

2 cups (500 ml) fresh shelled peas

4 sprigs fresh mint leaves

1 tablespoon (15 ml) lemon juice

- Heat olive oil in a medium saucepan. Add shallots and cook over medium heat for 1 minute or until soft.
- Add all but 2 tablespoons of the broth. Bring to a boil; reduce heat. Cover and simmer over medium-low heat for 4–5 minutes.
- Whisk cornstarch into the remaining 2 tablespoons of broth in a small bowl until smooth.
- Add cornstarch mixture into saucepan. Cook and stir until thickened, about 2 minutes.
- Stir in peas and mint. Let mixture cool slightly.
- Transfer pea mixture to a blender and blend until smooth. Transfer to a bowl and chill.
- To serve, stir in lemon juice, place in bowls and garnish with a bit of yogurt if desired, a thin slice of lemon peel and a sprig of fresh mint leaf.

Serves 4

Patty James Cooking School and Nutrition Centre for Grail Springs

Ginger Miso Soup

4 cups (1 L) water or vegetable broth

1 inch (2.5 cm) fresh ginger, grated or chopped

2 cloves fresh garlic, chopped

1 1/2 cups (375 ml) shitake mushrooms,
    stems removed and sliced

1 cup (250ml) Chinese cabbage, sliced thinly

1 bunch soba noodles

2 scallions, chopped

2 tablespoons (30 ml) chopped cilantro

1/2 teaspoon (2.5 ml) Sambal or red chili paste

Juice of 1 lime

2 tablespoons (30 ml) miso

- Combine everything but the miso in a stock pot and simmer until the soba noodles and the vegetables are cooked; about 10 minutes.
- Stir in the miso being careful not to let it boil.
- Taste for seasonings and if needed, add a splash of rice vinegar.

Serves 4

Roasted Garlic Soup

2 garlic bulbs
1 tablespoon (15 ml) olive oil
1 sliced onion
2 cloves fresh garlic, chopped
4 cups (1 L) water or vegetable broth
1/4 cup (50 ml) almond or rice milk
Himalayan salt to taste

- Cut the tops off the garlic bulbs, drizzle with olive oil and roast at 350F (180C) for about 40 minutes or until they become soft and golden.
- Remove from oven and let cool, then squeeze the cloves out of the peels.
- In a pot, sweat the onion and the fresh garlic until soft, add the roasted garlic and the water or broth.
- Simmer on low until the onions and fresh garlic are tender, about 20–30 minutes.
- Let cool slightly, then puree in a blender and strain through a mesh strainer.
- Return to the stove and bring back up to temperature.
- Whisk in the milk and season to taste.

Serves 4

Parsnip Soup

1 pound (450 g) parsnips, peeled and chopped

1 onion, sliced

2 cloves garlic

1/2 cup (125 ml) chopped leek

1 teaspoon coconut oil

4 cups (1 L) vegetable broth or water

1/2 cup (125 ml) almond or rice milk

Sea salt to taste

- Sweat parsnips, onion, garlic and leeks in coconut oil until soft, about 5 minutes.
- Add the broth or water and simmer for about 10–15 minutes.
- Let cool slightly and puree in a blender until smooth and strain through a mesh strainer.
- Return to the stove and bring back to heat.
- Add the milk and season with salt to your liking.

Serves 4

Parsnip & Apple Bisque

1 pound of organic parsnips, diced

2 ambrosia apples, chopped

1 carrot, chopped

1 celery stalk, diced

3 cloves garlic, minced

1 small red onion, diced

6 cups homemade veggie stock or 1 veggie bouillon cube
 & 6 cups water

1 tsp caraway seeds

pinch cinnamon

Himalayan salt to taste

1 tbsp olive oil

- In soup pot, sweat onions and garlic in olive oil on medium heat. Add carrot, celery and parsnip with salt, caraway and cinnamon. Add apple and stir.
- Cover with veggie stock (or water, and add veggie bouillon cube)
- Bring to a boil and simmer for 10 minutes. Turn down the heat and simmer until veggies are soft.
- Blend and adjust for consistency and taste.
- Serve garnished with fresh cilantro or finely chopped chives.

Serves 6

Power of Beets Borscht

Beets are powerful blood purifiers and cleansers, so much so that it's recommended to go easy on pure beet juice if doing a de-tox because it can flush out toxins very quickly, causing dizziness or light-headedness.

In this beautiful borscht, we use both the roots and the leaves. The leaves have even more nutrition than the roots, so when buying beets, don't throw them away!

You'll love the deep red colour of this soup, and your blood will sing with renewed vibrancy.

1 organic beet, diced

2 organic carrots, diced

1/2 red onion, diced

4 cloves of garlic, minced

2 celery stalks, diced

1 small zucchini, diced

2 or 3 beet leaves, sliced into fine ribbons

3 little buttercream potatoes or half a large one, diced

about 2 handfuls of red cabbage, sliced into ribbons

1 tbsp olive oil

2 tsp dill

Himalayan sea salt to taste

1 tsp caraway seeds

1 tbsp apple cider vinegar

1 tbsp agave nectar

- In a large soup pot, sautee onion and garlic until they sweat. Add carrots, celery, beets, potatoes, cabbage, caraway seeds and sea salt, and stir.
- Cover veggies with water or homemade veggie broth and bring to a boil. Turn down and simmer until beets and potatoes are soft.
- Add zucchini and beet greens, and a pinch more caraway seeds if desired, and simmer a few more minutes.
- Turn off the heat and add dill, agave nectar and apple cider vinegar. Taste and adjust seasoning to your liking.
- This soup is nice served with a dollop of Raw Nut "Cream".

Serves 2

Butternut Squash & Fennel Soup

As soon as squash and fennel begin to appear at the market in fall, you've got two very flavourful, nutrient-dense ingredients that combine beautifully for an outstandingly rich and creamy blended soup. It's velvety smooth, sweet, soothing and super comforting.

1 tbsp olive oil or coconut oil

5 or 6 cloves garlic, minced

1 medium red onion, diced

1 medium carrot, diced

2 stalks celery, diced

1 organic medium butternut squash, peeled and chopped

1 fennel bulb, washed and diced from bulb to leaf

1 veggie bouillon cube & water or 6 cups of homemade
   veggie broth

Himalayan sea salt to taste

Splash of maple syrup to taste

2 tsp "nanami togarashi"

- In a large soup pot, sautee onions and garlic in a little olive or coconut oil until they sweat. Add carrot and celery.
- Meanwhile, peel and chop your squash, then toss into the mix. Add fennel and stir.
- Cover the veggies with water or broth and turn heat to almost high. Throw in one or two cubes of veggie bouillon if not using homemade broth, and bring to a boil, then turn down the heat and let simmer for 45 minutes to an hour.

- Turn off the heat, add a splash of maple syrup, some sea salt to taste, and if you have access to a Japanese market, this wonderful condiment called "nanami togarashi" is the secret ingredient for this soup. It's a blend of chilis, black sesame, seaweed and citrus, and I find it gives this creamy, sweet and licoricy soup a wonderful hint of exotic spice.
- Blend the soup with an immersion blender or in a food processor until smooth, and adjust the seasoning to your liking.

Serves 6

Marinated Tofu Salad

2 1/2 cups (625 ml) tofu, cut into cubes

1 head of lettuce, leaves separated

2 tomatoes, cut into wedges

1/2 cup (125 ml) sprouts

2 carrots, sliced

1 tablespoon (15 ml) sesame seeds, toasted

Marinade

4 tablespoons (60 ml) Bragg liquid amino

2 teaspoons (10 ml) olive oil

1/2 teaspoon (2.5 ml) chopped fresh ginger

1 tablespoon (15 ml) lemon juice

- Combine marinade ingredients in a bowl.
- Add tofu and toss to coat. Marinate for 10–15 minutes.
- Combine lettuce leaves, tomatoes, sprouts and carrots in a bowl.
- Drain tofu. Reserve marinade.
- Add tofu to salad. Toss. Scatter with sesame seeds.
- Just before serving, drizzle with remaining marinade.

Serves 4

Asparagus and Salmon Salad

20 asparagus spears
Assorted lettuce leaves
8 smoked salmon slices

Lemon Yogurt Dressing
1 cup (250 ml) organic low fat yogurt
1 tablespoon (15 ml) freshly squeezed lemon juice
1 teaspoon (5 ml) chopped lemon zest
1 tablespoon (15 ml) chopped dill
1 teaspoon (5 ml) ground cumin

- Combine yogurt, lemon zest and juice, dill and cumin.
- Steam the asparagus until tender but still crisp. Chill in the refrigerator.
- Wash and arrange lettuce leaves on a serving plate.
- Roll up each salmon slice and arrange with asparagus on top.
- Drizzle dressing over salad and serve.

Serves 4

Basil, Orange, and Peach Salad

1 cup (250 ml) fresh basil leaves
6 organic oranges, peeled, sliced
3 peaches, peeled, sliced
1 red onion, sliced

Apple and Garlic Dressing

1 garlic clove, crushed
2 tablespoons (30 ml) red wine vinegar
2 tablespoons (30 ml) apple cider vinegar
2 tablespoons (30 ml) safflower oil

- Arrange basil leaves on a platter. Set aside.
- Toss together oranges, peaches and onion in a bowl.
- Combine garlic, vinegars, and oil.
- Drizzle over orange mixture. Toss.
- Arrange orange and peach mixture on top of basil leaves.
- Serve immediately.

Serves 4

Broccoli, Tomato, and Watercress Salad

2 cups (500 ml) broccoli, chopped

2 cups (500 ml) cherry tomatoes

1 bunch watercress, stems removed, coarsely chopped

1 1/2 teaspoons (7.5 ml) red wine vinegar

1 tablespoon (15 ml) olive oil or flax oil

1/2 teaspoon (2.5 ml) garlic, minced

1/2 teaspoon (2.5 ml) Himalayan salt

- Place water in a medium saucepan and bring to a boil.
- Add broccoli and cook for 1 1/2 minutes.
- Drain broccoli and plunge into ice water to cool.
  It should still be crisp.
- In a large bowl combine the broccoli, tomatoes and watercress.
- In a small bowl whisk together the vinegar, oil, garlic, and salt to taste.
- Drizzle over vegetables and toss to coat.
  Serve immediately.

Serves 4

Serving ideas: The serving size here is approximately 1/2 cup as a side, however it is very low in calories so feel free to serve it on lettuce or double the portion size and serve with chicken or fish for lunch. You could also add garbanzo beans if you like.

Patty James Cooking School and Nutrition Centre for Grail Springs

Arame Salad

1³/4 oz (50 g) arame strips (dried seaweed)

1 red pepper, diced

1 bunch scallions, diced

2 tablespoons (30 ml) rice vinegar

2 teaspoons (10 ml) toasted sesame oil

1 tablespoon (15 ml) sesame seeds, toasted

- Soak the arame for 15 minutes in cold water and drain well.
- Combine vinegar and toasted sesame oil.
- Toss in the arame and vegetables.
- Sprinkle with toasted sesame seeds. Serve immediately.

Serves 8

Serving option: Sprinkle with Gomashio (toasted sesame and Himalayan salt. See page 150.)

Patty James Cooking School and Nutrition Centre for Grail Springs

Crispy Sesame Tofu

3 tablespoons (45 ml) olive oil

3 tablespoons (45 ml) tamari soy sauce

3 tablespoons (45 ml) ginger, grated

8 cloves garlic, minced

1/2 teaspoon (2.5 ml) crushed red pepper

1 pound (455 g) tofu, extra firm

3 tablespoons (45 ml) sesame seeds

- Combine all ingredients except tofu and sesame seeds in a bowl to make a marinade and mix well.
- Slice the tofu into 1/2-inch strips and arrange in a baking dish. Pour marinade over top.
- Marinate for about an hour in the refrigerator, turning once.
- Preheat oven to 400F.
- Press sesame seeds into tofu.
- Bake uncovered for 25 minutes (or longer for crisper tofu), turning once.

Serves 4

Serving ideas: This is wonderful served on a spinach salad. Dress the spinach with a miso dressing and toss with thin slices of red onion, mushrooms, and sunflower sprouts. Top with the warm tofu and serve.

This is also a great filling in pita bread or wrapped in a tortilla with lettuce, avocado and sliced tomatoes.

Patty James Cooking School and Nutrition Centre for Grail Springs

Watermelon and Mango Salad with Citrus Dressing

5 cups (1250 ml) watermelon, seeded and cubed

1 1/2 cups (375 ml) mango, cubed

3 tablespoons (45 ml) orange juice, fresh

2 teaspoons (10 ml) lime zest

1 tablespoon (15 ml) lime juice

2 teaspoons (10 ml) maple syrup

6 mint leaves, sliced

- Combine watermelon and mango in a large bowl.
- Combine orange juice, zest, lime juice, and maple syrup, stirring with a whisk.
- Drizzle over fruit mixture; toss gently to coat.
- Sprinkle with mint.

Serves: 4

Serving ideas: Makes a great mid-morning snack.

Patty James Cooking School and Nutrition Centre for Grail Springs

Southwestern Caesar Salad

2 hearts romaine lettuce, washed and dried

1 clove garlic

1/2 lemon, juiced

1/2 teaspoon (2.5 ml) Dijon mustard

1 teaspoon (5 ml) chili powder, divided

1/3 cup (75 ml) olive oil, divided

3 tortillas

1/4 cup (50 ml) organic white cheddar cheese, grated

1/2 tomato, sliced

1/4 cup (50 ml) raw pumpkin seeds, roasted

1/2 avocado, sliced (optional – adds 40 extra calories
   but also adds "good" fat)

- Chop and place the romaine lettuce in a large salad bowl. Place in refrigerator.
- Whisk together the garlic, lemon juice, Dijon and 1/2 teaspoon chili powder in a small bowl. Continue whisking while you pour in half of the olive oil in a thin stream.
- Cut tortillas into thin strips and toss with remaining olive oil and remaining chili powder. Bake at 350F for 15–20 minutes or until golden brown. Remove and put aside.
- Dress the salad and toss well. Garnish with tomatoes, cheese, pumpkin seeds, tortillas strips, and avocado. Toss again and serve immediately.

Serves 4

Patty James Cooking School and Nutrition Centre for Grail Springs

Warm Chickpea Salad

For the Vinaigrette

1 teaspoon (5 ml) grainy mustard

1/4 cup (50 ml) apple cider vinegar

1/2 cup (125 ml) grape seed or other oil

Juice of 1 lemon

1 clove garlic, minced

1 shallot minced

Himalayan salt and cayenne pepper to taste

For the salad

2 cups (500 ml) cooked organic chickpeas

1 carrot, diced

1 onion, diced

1 zucchini, diced

1 head of broccoli, cut into florets

1 red pepper, diced

1 teaspoon (5 ml) cumin

1 tablespoon (15 ml) curry powder

- Combine vinaigrette ingredients and set aside.
- Sweat the vegetables until tender in a large pot.
- Add the curry and cumin; stir until it starts to toast.
- Toss in the cooked chickpeas and pour in the vinaigrette, heating until warm.
- Season with Himalayan salt and cayenne pepper to taste.
- Serve with fresh watercress or arugula.

Serves 2–4

Mediterranean Quinoa Salad

Quinoa was the "gold of the Incas" because of the energy it supplied their warriors. Yes, if you've got quinoa in your pantry, you're wealthy. This superfood is actually a seed, but cooks up quickly like a grain and has a really nice sort of creamy, mildly nutty flavour. I love cooking with quinoa because of its pure speed. You can make up a pot in about 15 minutes.

To cook quinoa, wash and rinse first, then cover 2-1 with water, bring to a boil, then turn down to minimum and cook, covered for 15 minutes. For this recipe, for 2, try cooking one and a half cups of quinoa with 3 cups of water. It will expand and yield 3 cups or so of quinoa.

3 cups quinoa, cooked

1/2 cup organic chick peas, soaked overnight and cooked
   (or half a can of organic chick peas)

5 sundried tomatoes, chopped

half a cup of hulled hemp seeds

half a Persian or English cucumber, diced

2 tbsp capers

3 large spicy olives, pitted and chopped

half a cup of toasted pine nuts

1 organic lemon, juiced

drizzle extra virgin olive oil

Himalayan crystal salt to taste

- Mix everything together in a bowl, then drizzle with fresh squeezed lemon juice and extra virgin olive oil, and add salt to taste.

Serves 2

Sacred Millet Salad

Millet was considered a sacred crop by the ancient Chinese. It contains no gluten, so those with wheat allergies can use it as a nutritious substitute grain. Millet is healing on the stomach, it's alkaline and retains its alkalinity when cooked. It's loaded with B vitamins, namely niacin and B6, calcium and other minerals, and is mildly nutty in flavour.

To prepare millet, about 2 to 1 water to grain will do it. Wash and rinse the millet first, then add water and bring to a boil. Turn down the heat to low and leave covered for about 20 minutes.

2 cups cooked millet

1 package Morning Star veggie "Chik'n" Strips or Yves Veggie "Chicken" Tenders

1 long English cucumber, diced

1 red pepper, cored and diced

1 carrot, diced

1 green onion, chopped

handful of toasted sesame seeds

handful of tamari-roasted sunflower seeds

Asian Dressing

2 tbsp tamari

2 tbsp toasted sesame oil

juice of 1 lime

juice of 1 lemon

1 tsp fresh grated ginger

1tbsp maple syrup

- Toss the "Chik'n" Strips in a skillet on medium-high heat with some sesame oil, a splash of tamari and a splash of maple syrup. Stir until the edges brown and "Chik'n" is heated through.
- Toss all ingredients into a large stainless steel bowl and mix through. Serve on a bed of baby spinach topped with the Asian Dressing and garnished with toasted sesame seeds or tamari-roasted sunflower seeds.

Serves 6

Dolmas with Goat Feta and Cranberries

1 cup (250 ml) brown rice, short grain

2 cups (500 ml) water

1 bunch collard greens, 6 medium leaves

1/2 cup (125 ml) almonds, dry toasted, finely chopped

1/3 cup (75 ml) cranberries, dried, sliced in half

1/2 cup (125 ml) goat feta cheese

1/2 teaspoon (2.5 ml) Himalayan salt

1/2 teaspoon (2.5 ml) lemon zest

1/4 teaspoon (0.625 ml) rosemary, ground

- Combine rice and water in a large pot and bring to a boil. Reduce heat, cover and simmer on low heat for 45 minutes or until done.
- Meanwhile, wash collard greens and then blanch for 30 seconds. Cool and set aside.
- When rice is slightly cooled, stir in almonds, salt and seasonings, cranberries and feta cheese.
- Gently cut large stems from collard leaves. Lay a collard leaf flat on a cutting board and place a scoopful of the rice mixture in the centre of the leaf. Roll up like a burrito, tucking in the sides of the leaf. Repeat for all leaves.
- To reheat, place in a steamer, over boiling water and warm for 5 minutes. Garnish with orange-infused olive oil or orange or grapefruit juice and serve.

Serves 6

Serving ideas: Serve for lunch with a spring mix and flower petal salad with a lemon vinaigrette. Garnish the dolmas with a twist of orange.

Patty James Cooking School and Nutrition Centre for Grail Springs

Beet in a Blanket

Not only is this beautiful on a plate with a side of organic greens, it's a loaded lunch that'll give you energy and stamina while still feeling light and fresh in the body.

1 ripe avocado

1/4 package soft "silken" tofu

1 tbsp Braggs Amino Acids (or more to taste)

1 small beet, grated

1 carrot, grated

handful of organic salad greens

1 tbsp apple cider vinegar

1 tbsp tahini

2 10-inch sprouted grain wraps or spinach or sundried tomato
  tortilla wraps

- Mash avocado with a fork. Add tofu and continue blending until smooth. Add Bragg's Aminos. Taste and add another splash of Bragg's if desired.
- Lay out flour tortillas and spread tofu mixture to about 1 inch from edges.
- Toss greens with a splash of apple cider vinegar.
- Layer beets, carrots and greens. Careful not to layer too heavily or tortilla will be difficult to roll and stick. It might take a bit of practice.
- Roll up tortilla, spread a little tahini on the edges to stick it together, then cut on the diagonal into two halves.

Serves 2

Mains

California Girl Roasted Root Veggie Sushi

1 cup cooked short grain organic brown rice (cooked with a little
   more water than usual to make it sticky)

1 carrot, thinly sliced on the diagonal

1 small yam, thinly sliced on the diagonal

1 small red onion, finely sliced into slivers

1/4 butternut squash, thinly sliced on the diagonal

1 or 2 tsp garlic powder

1 tbsp olive oil

2 tsp Himalayan sea salt

handful of organic salad greens

3 or 4 shiitake mushrooms, sliced

4 sushi nori sheets (available at health food stores and
   Asian markets)

wasabi (be sure to get pure wasabi with no artificial colouring
   or msg)

sushi ginger (available at health food stores and Asian markets,
   again, get pure-not artificially coloured ginger)

tamari for dipping

splash maple syrup

1 tbsp agave nectar

1 tbsp rice vinegar

toasted sesame seeds, cilantro for garnish

- When brown rice is cooked, transfer it to a large stainless steel bowl and add a splash of agave nectar, a splash of rice vinegar and a pinch of Himalayan sea salt. Mix together and allow to cool. Rice should be nice and sticky, slightly sweet.
- Roast root veggies with sea salt and garlic powder on a lightly olive-oiled cookie sheet in a 350-degree oven for 45 minutes, stirring several times throughout.
- While veggies are in oven, toss shiitake mushrooms into a skillet on med-high with a splash of tamari and a splash of maple syrup. Cook until tender.
- Take veggies out of oven and cool.
- Both rice and veggies should be cooled to room temperature before you begin working with the nori.
- Place a sushi nori sheet on a bamboo sushi mat. With a wooden spoon or your hands, place a thin layer of sticky brown rice on a piece of sushi nori. With wet fingers, work rice out towards edges, leaving about a centimeter around the edges.
- Layer greens, roasted veggies and shiitake mushrooms across the middle of the roll.
- Beginning with the edge closest to you, carefully roll up the sushi away from you. When the sushi roll is complete, squeeze tightly around sushi mat to ensure it stays in one piece.
- Wet a sharp knife and slice sushi roll into 8 pieces. Arrange nicely on a plate with some edible flowers, sushi ginger, some dipping tamari and a bit of wasabi.
- Sprinkle the entire plate with toasted or black sesame seeds and garnish with fresh cilantro.

Yield: 4 rolls

Chickpea Croquettes

This is an easy, healthy lunch or dinner you can make in minutes if you have canned organic chickpeas on hand. If you're organized, though, soaking chickpeas overnight and cooking them up is even better.

1 cup organic chick peas, washed & soaked overnight then
    cooked, or 1 can organic chick peas, drained and rinsed
1/2 cup organic cornmeal
2 cloves garlic, minced
1/4 medium red onion, finely diced
1 small zucchini, finely grated
1 tsp each, cumin seeds, coriander powder, curry powder
1/2 tsp Himalayan sea salt
1 tsp coconut oil

- Blend drained and cooked chickpeas in cuisinart, or mash with a fork if you prefer a slightly chunkier consistency.
- In a large bowl, combine all ingredients. Depending how much water your zucchini contains, you may have to add a splash of spring water for a slightly wet consistency. Form into patties about the size of your palm.
- In a cast iron frying pan, heat coconut oil on medium. Cook patties for about 10 minutes on each side.

Serve with Mango Chutney and a side of organic greens for a complete meal.

Sweet Yellow Pepper Gazpacho

On a warm summer evening when you feel like something elegant and light, try this chilled soup filled with fresh-picked goodness of the season.

2 lbs ripe organic roma tomatoes
1 long English cucumber, peeled
1 sweet red onion
3 ripe yellow peppers, cored
4 cloves fresh garlic, chopped
3 tbsp cold pressed virgin olive oil
2 tbsp apple cider vinegar
small bunch fresh basil
small bunch fresh parsley
1 sprig fresh thyme
2 tsp Himalayan sea salt
fresh pepper to taste

- Remove skins from tomatoes by briefly plunging them into boiling water. Dice and blend in a cuisinart until smooth.
- Coarsely chop the rest of the ingredients and add to the cuisinart. Pulse a few times to blend, but not puree.
- Adjust seasoning with salt, pepper and chopped fresh herbs.
- Garnish with a basil or parsley sprig, and serve chilled with a side of Sacred Millet Salad.

Yield: 6 appetizers

Ginger "Veggie Beef" & Buckwheat

With a little help from our friends at Gardein™, who make plant-based "chicken and beef" products for Yves and Morningstar, now available in your grocery store, this wonderful warming Asian stir-fry can be prepared in 5 minutes.

It can be made with whatever veggies you have in the fridge, and topped with cashews, sesame, black sesame, sunflower, or any other seed or nut you happen to have on hand.

Ginger is great for the stomach and enhances appetite and digestion, as well as improving assimilation and transportation of nutrients to the appropriate body cells. It's also a cardiotonic (good for the heart), and is widely used therapeutically in India for joint pain and circulatory problems. So be liberal with the ginger...It's medicine!

2 portions of 100% organic buckwheat noodles
    (available at health food stores or Asian markets)

3 or 4 cloves garlic, minced

1 tsp sambal oelek (red chili paste)

2 or 3 tbsp fresh grated ginger

1 tbsp toasted sesame oil

2 tbsp tamari

1 tbsp maple syrup

5 or 6 shiitake mushrooms, sliced

1 celery stalk, cut on the diagonal

1 carrot, cut on the diagonal

half a zucchini, cut into half-moons

half a red pepper, julienned

a handful of broccoli florets

1 package Morningstar Farms Veggie Steak Strips
    (or Yves Veggie Beef Tenders)

- Prep everything before you begin so you can just add to the pan and toss.
- Boil water and cook buckwheat noodles for 5 minutes or until al dente. Note that 100% buckwheat noodles will cook more quickly than wheat noodles, so check on them after just a few minutes.
- In a wok or large frying pan on medium-high, sautee garlic, chili paste and ginger in sesame oil. Add shiitake mushrooms and toss quickly. Add celery and carrot and stir.
- Add a splash of tamari. Continue stirring quickly and add broccoli, zucchini, red pepper and "beef". Add another splash of tamari if veggies begin to stick to pan.
- When the broccoli has turned bright green and the veggies are cooked to your liking, turn off the heat and add a tiny splash of maple syrup.
- Strain the noodles and make a nest on 2 plates. Top with ginger "beef" & veggies and sprinkle your favourite seed or nut on top. (I like black sesame seeds with this recipe.)

Serves 2

Chilly Day Chili

Nothing warms body and soul better than a hearty bowl of vegetarian chili.

1 cup organic black beans, washed and soaked overnight

1 can organic crushed or diced tomatoes (or ? pound of fresh ripe organic tomatoes, diced)

1/2 cup of organic millet

1 carrot, diced

1 celery stalk, diced

4 cloves garlic, minced

1 onion, diced

1 tbsp olive oil

1tsp (or so) each, cumin seeds, cumin powder, oregano, basil, chili paste (sambal oelek),

1 tbsp organic cocoa powder

2 tbsp chili powder

splash apple cider vinegar

1 tbsp agave nectar

1 tsp or so sea salt

1 bay leaf

small bunch of cilantro

- Rinse soaking beans and cover again with water in a large soup pot. Add a bay leaf and bring to a boil. Simmer until they're cooked (about half an hour).
- Meanwhile, sautee garlic and onion in a little olive oil in a large frying pan. Stir until they sweat, then add carrots and celery.

- Add spices and stir. Add a splash of water if it's too dry.
- Add veggies and spices to the cooked black beans, along with can of tomatoes and rinsed millet. You may have to add some more water here depending on how much is left from cooking the beans.
- Add sea salt, a splash of apple cider vinegar and a dollop of agave nectar.
- Simmer until millet is cooked and allow chili to sit as long as possible before eating. It's even better the next day.
- Sprinkle with chopped fresh cilantro and serve with a dollop of Raw Nut "Cream".

Serves 4

Quinoa & Kale Stuffed Tomatoes

This dish looks elegant on a plate and is a beautiful, light and healthy meal to serve to guests.

1 large organic heirloom tomato, cored
1 cup of quinoa, cooked
1/2 cup of broccoli florets
4 dinosaur kale leaves, cut into fine ribbons
1/4 red onion, finely diced
3 cloves garlic, minced
splash tamari
Himalayan sea salt
1tbsp olive oil

- Cook quinoa with spring water (2 to 1) and a pinch of sea salt, first rinsing it well in a fine sieve.
- In a cast iron fry pan, heat olive oil and sautee garlic, onion, broccoli and kale. When the broccoli and kale have turned a nice dark green, add a splash of tamari, stir through and remove from heat.
- When quinoa is cooked (10 or 15 minutes), add it to the veggies and mix through. (You decide how much.)
- Hollow out the center of a large organic tomato and add the mixture. It's good to go here, or you may wish to pop it in the oven for ten minutes to cook the tomato and heat it through.

Serve with the rest of the veggie-quinoa mix on the side and drizzle with raw nut "cream".

Serves 1

Power Patties

These patties are loaded in grain, legume, seed and nut protein, and will give you all the clean, balanced energy you need to get through the day.

1 cup short grain organic brown rice
1 cup organic green lentils
1/4 red onion, diced
1 cup walnuts, chopped
1/2 cup pumpkin seeds
1 tbsp tahini
1/2 cup nutritional yeast
1 tsp each, basil, rosemary, sage and oregano
Himalayan sea salt to taste

- Cook brown rice and lentils in separate pots, each with a little more than 2 cups of water. (We're aiming for a slightly sticky consistency so the rice and lentils will stick together.)
- Combine all ingredients in a large bowl and taste. Adjust seasoning to your liking and form into patties.
- Bake on a lightly oiled cookie sheet at 300 for about 15 minutes on each side.
- You can finish them on the stovetop grill, browning them on each side, or simply bake a little longer and they're good to go.
- Serve drizzled with Tahini-Garlic Sauce and a side of organic greens for a complete meal.

Serves 4

Salmon en Papillote

4 6-oz (180 g) salmon fillets, skin removed,
    washed and dried
4 tablespoons (60 ml) lemon juice
2 teaspoons (10 ml) toasted sesame oil
2 teaspoons (10 ml) ginger, freshly grated
2 teaspoons (10 ml) Himalayan salt
1 red pepper, quartered
4 cups (1 L) spinach leaves
12 stalks asparagus

- Mix the lemon juice, toasted sesame oil, ginger, salt and pepper in a small bowl.
- Place washed and dried spinach leaves down the centre of an 18-inch-long piece of parchment paper.
- Place the salmon atop the leaves and arrange the asparagus and red pepper on top of the salmon. Drizzle with the oil mixture.
- Bring up both ends of the parchment paper and fold; crimp edges to close tightly. Place on a baking sheet and baked at 375F for 25 minutes.

Serves 4

Serving ideas: You may open at the table if you like, but be cautious of the steam when it is released. Serve with a tossed green salad. You may also substitute the salmon with any kind of fish, tofu, or pounded chicken breast (bake chicken for 30 minutes).

Patty James Cooking School and Nutrition Centre for Grail Springs

Orange Roughy with Ginger Sesame Marinade

4 orange roughy fillets

Marinade

1/2 cup (125 ml) rice wine vinegar

1/4 cup (50 ml) water

1/4 cup (50 ml) yellow miso

1/4 cup (50 ml) green onion, chopped

2 tablespoons (30 ml) maple syrup

2 tablespoons (30 ml) fresh ginger, peeled and minced

2 tablespoons (30 ml) low sodium soy sauce

4 teaspoons (20 ml) olive oil

2 teaspoons (10 ml) dark sesame oil

- Mix marinade ingredients together and marinate the fillets for approximately one hour.
- Drain and discard marinade and grill fillets for approximately 4–5 minutes per side.

Serves 4

Serving ideas: Also makes a delicious marinade for any type of white fish, chicken or tofu.

Try the marinade with tempeh: Slice tempeh into 1/2-inch slices. Steam tempeh for 15 minutes. Drain and place in a bowl. Pour the marinade over the tempeh and let sit for one hour. Grill or sauté for 5 minutes each side. Serve with a cabbage slaw and buckwheat noodles cooked in miso-flavoured water.

Patty James Cooking School and Nutrition Centre for Grail Springs

Salsa Borracha on Red Snapper

4 red snapper fillets

Juice of 1 lime

2 pasilla peppers, dried

1 chipotle pepper, dried

1 1/2 cups (375 ml) water

3 cloves garlic

1/4 cup (50 ml) olive oil

1 jalapeno pepper, fresh

1/2 cup (125 ml) tequila

1 large onion, coarsely chopped

1 1/2 teaspoon (7.5 ml) Himalayan salt

1 tablespoon (15 ml) red wine vinegar

- Marinate fillets in lime juice and olive oil. Set aside.
- Place the dried peppers in a non-oiled pan and toast for 1–2 minutes on each side.
- Remove from heat and remove stems and seeds. Place in a bowl and soak in water from about an hour.
- Drain peppers, saving 1/2 cup (125 ml) of the liquid (save the rest for another use.)
- Place the peppers, the liquid, and the remaining ingredients in a food processor or blender and puree until smooth.
- Grill the red snapper to taste and top with salsa.

Serves 4

Serving ideas: This sauce is delicious on many different fishes. Or, serve with red or black beans that you have soaked overnight and cooked with a piece of kombu seaweed (to make them more digestible and to add minerals), and a wedge of lime.

Patty James Cooking School and Nutrition Centre for Grail Springs

Poached Lemongrass Red Snapper with Quinoa

Quinoa

4 cups (1 L) purified water

2 organic vegetable bouillon cubes

2 cups (500 ml) quinoa, rinsed thoroughly

- Bring water to a boil. Add bouillon and quinoa.
- Reduce to simmer for 20 minutes or until quinoa is tender. Set aside.

Red Snapper

4 stalks of lemongrass split lengthwise

2 cups (500 ml) purified water

8 4-oz (120 g) pieces of red snapper

1 pound (455 g) organic baby spinach, blanched

- Add lemongrass to water and bring to boil.
- Remove from heat and let cool overnight.
- Reheat to simmer. Add red snapper and cover with lid.
- Remove from heat and let sit for 15 minutes.
- Serve with quinoa and blanched spinach.

Serves 8

Miso Marinated Salmon

1/4 cup (50 ml) miso paste

2 tablespoons (30 ml) maple syrup

2 tablespoons (30 ml) rice wine vinegar

1 tablespoon (15 ml) olive oil

4 6-oz (170 g) skinless salmon fillets

1/3 cup (75 ml) fresh lime juice

2 tablespoons (30 ml) minced peeled fresh ginger

1 tablespoon (15 ml) black sesame seeds, toasted with
   a sprinkle of Himalayan salt

- Combine first 4 ingredients in a small bowl.
- Brush fish with the miso mixture. Cover and chill
  30 minutes.
- Combine lime juice and ginger in a small saucepan
  over medium heat, and bring to a boil.
- When it has reached a boil, turn off the heat and set aside.
- Preheat broiler or grill.
- Place the fish on a broiler rack and broil for 3 minutes
  on each side or until the fish flakes easily when tested
  with a fork.
- Drizzle the lime mixture over the fish. Sprinkle with the
  toasted sesame seeds.

Serves 4

Ginger and Green Onion Tilapia

You can replace tilapia with salmon, bass, pickerel, pike or any fish that steams or poaches well. You can even use this for chicken.

Marinade

1/2 cup (125 ml) Bragg liquid aminos

1 1/2 teaspoons (7.5 ml) pure maple syrup

Juice of 1/2 a lime, plus the zest

2 tablespoons (30 ml) rice wine vinegar

1 tablespoon (15 ml) toasted sesame oil

4 tilapia filets

2-inch piece fresh ginger, cut into matchsticks

2–3 fresh green onions, slivered

- Preheat oven to 375F.
- Combine Bragg, maple syrup, lime juice and zest, vinegar, and oil and set aside.
- Oil a baking dish with grape seed oil then lay out the fish and add enough of the marinade sauce to come 1/3 up the thickness of the fish.
- Cooking time will vary depending on the thickness of the fish. Check every 5 minutes to preference.
- Plate fish over black or red wild rice and cover with green onion and ginger, then ladle warm sauce over fish. Serve with bright steamed or grilled vegetables.

Serves 4

Pecan Crusted Chicken with Mustard Sauce

4 6-oz (180 g) chicken breasts, pounded

2 tablespoons (30 ml) rice flour

4 tablespoons (60 ml) pecans

1 teaspoon (5 ml) thyme

1 1/2 teaspoons (7.5 ml) paprika

1 teaspoon (5 ml) Himalayan salt

2 dashes cayenne pepper

2 eggs

2 tablespoons water

Yogurt sauce

1 cup (250 ml) plain yogurt

2 tablespoons (30 ml) Dijon mustard

1 tablespoon (15 ml) rice vinegar

1/2 teaspoon (2.5 ml) maple syrup

- In a food processor, pulse the pecans with the rice flour, thyme, paprika, salt, pepper and cayenne. Transfer to a mixing bowl.
- Whisk together the eggs and water in a small bowl.
- Dip each chicken breast in the egg mixture and then into the nut mixture. Let dry on bakers rack for a few minutes.
- Bake for 30 minutes at 375F.
- Combine the yogurt and remaining ingredients in a small saucepan. Heat only until warm.
- To serve, pour sauce over chicken.

Serves 4

Patty James Cooking School and Nutrition Centre for Grail Springs

Cucumber and Feta Salsa
with Grilled Chicken

1/2 cup (125 ml) goat feta cheese, crumbled

2 tablespoons (30 ml) lemon juice

3 tablespoons (45 ml) olive oil

1/4 teaspoon (1.25 ml) Himalayan salt

3/4 cup (175 ml) cucumber, seeded and diced

1/2 cup (125 ml) red onion, diced

2 tablespoons (30 ml) fresh mint, minced

2 tablespoons (30 ml) fresh dill, minced

1 pound (455 g) chicken breast, grilled and
   thinly sliced

8 cups (2 L) lettuce leaves, use spring mix or mesclun mix

- Marinate the chicken breast in 2 tablespoons of olive oil, 1 tablespoon of lemon juice, and salt for approximately one hour.
- Grill or bake chicken and let cool, then thinly slice and set aside.
- For the salsa, combine the feta, and remaining lemon juice and oil, and mash with a fork until crumbly. Add the cucumber, onion, mint and dill.
- Place chicken slices atop 2 cups lettuce mix per person and top with approximately 6 tablespoons of salsa. Garnish with a lemon or lime wedge.

Serves 4

Patty James Cooking School and Nutrition Centre for Grail Springs

South American Vegetarian Stew

2 cups (500 ml) carrot juice (freshly juiced)

1 tablespoon (15 ml) olive oil

1/2 cup (125 ml) onion, coarsely chopped

2 cloves garlic, coarsely chopped

3/4 cup (175 ml) shitake mushrooms, sliced

3 cups (750 ml) tomato juice, (if using canned use
    low sodium)

2 1/4 teaspoons (11.25 ml) chilli powder

1 cup (250 ml) yams, peeled and chopped into
    1/2-inch cubes

1/4 cup (50 ml) quinoa, thoroughly rinsed

3/4 cup (175 ml) zucchini, 1-inch slices
    (or other seasonal vegetables)

1 cup (250 ml) kidney beans, cooked

3/4 cup (175 ml) corn (fresh preferable)

Lemon juice to taste

- Heat oil in a large, heavy pot and sauté onions, garlic and mushrooms for about 5 minutes.
- Add tomato and carrot juices, chili powder, yams and quinoa and bring to a boil. Reduce heat to a simmer, cover and cook for about 10–15 minutes.
- Just as the yams are beginning to become tender, add zucchini. Simmer covered until vegetables are all tender, about 10 minutes more.
- Add the beans and corn, cook until heated through. Season to taste with fresh lemon juice.

Serves 6

Serving ideas: Each serving is about 2 cups (500 ml). Serve with a mixed green salad with a lemon vinaigrette, which brings out the flavour of the carrots nicely. You may leave out the yams and add other seasonal vegetables such as baby spinach leaves; place the baby leaves in the bottom of the bowl and pour the hot stew over the top. Garnish with a topping of fresh yogurt and a curled lemon rind.

Patty James Cooking School and Nutrition Centre for Grail Springs

Sides, Sauces, and Snacks

Braised Fennel with Orange and Walnuts

1 bulb fennel, cored, quartered and sliced

3 shallots, sliced

1 tablespoon (15 ml) coconut oil

1 clove garlic, minced

1 cup (250 ml) freshly squeezed orange juice

1/4 teaspoon (0.625 ml) Himalayan salt

1/4 cup (50 ml) walnuts

- Sweat the shallots with the fennel in the coconut oil.
- Add the garlic and orange juice and cover on low heat for approximately 10 minutes or until tender and most of the juice has absorbed.
- Season with salt, add walnuts, and serve.

Serves: 4–6

Red Rice Stuffing

3 tablespoons (45 ml) grape seed oil

1/2 cup (125 ml) celery, chopped

1/2 cup (125 ml) carrot, diced

3/4 cup (175 ml) onion, diced

2 cloves garlic, minced

2 cups (500 ml) Himalayan red rice

4 cups (1 L) vegetable stock

1/2 piece kombu

1/4 cup (50 ml) chopped pitted dates

1/2 cup (125 ml) dried cranberries

1/2 cup (125 ml) chopped Gala apple

1/4 cup (50 ml) raisins

2 teaspoons (10 ml) Himalayan salt

2 tablespoons (30 ml) fresh chopped sage

1 tablespoon (15 ml) fresh chopped thyme

- Over medium heat sweat the vegetables in the grape seed oil and add the rice, stirring until covered with the oil.
- Add the stock and the kombu and let come to a simmer.
- Cover until stock is mostly absorbed and then add the rest of the ingredients.
- Cover again until rice is tender.

Yield: approx 6 cups stuffing

Dijon Sweet Potatoes

2 medium to large sweet potatoes or yams

2 tablespoons (30 ml) roasted garlic

2 teaspoon (10 ml) Dijon mustard

1 tablespoon (15 ml) organic yogurt

1/2 teaspoon (2.5 ml) Himalayan salt

- Bake sweet potato in a 350F (180C) oven for
  40–50 minutes until soft.
- While still hot, peel (wear oven mitts!) and run through
  a food mill.
- Add roasted garlic, mustard, yogurt and salt. Mix well
  and taste.
- If necessary adjust seasoning.

Serves 4

Serving idea: For a Tex-Mex flair add 1 teaspoon (5 ml) ground
cumin seed and a pinch of cayenne pepper.

Braised Radishes and Apples

2 bunches fresh radishes
1 Gala apple (or other firm textured)
1 tablespoon (15 ml) shallots, sliced
$1/2$ cup (125 ml) apple cider
Pinch Himalayan salt
1 teaspoon (5 ml) grape seed oil

- Chop apples into $1/2$-inch wedges.
- Trim the radish ends off and cut in half.
- Add the oil to a small pot on medium heat and add the shallots to slightly sweat.
- Add the radishes and apples and sweat for 2 minutes, then add the apple cider and salt.
- Cover and let braise on low to medium heat until tender and the juice had reduced to a glaze, about 2 tablespoons.

Serves 4

Healthy Cheeseless Cheese Dip

2 cups (500 ml) cashews

1 cup (250 ml) red pepper, chopped

1 tablespoon (15 ml) toasted sesame oil

3 tablespoons (45 ml) nutritional yeast

Himalayan salt to taste

3/4 cup (175 ml) water

Juice of 1 lemon

- Combine all ingredients in a blender until smooth.
  It will thicken as it cools.

Serving ideas: Wonderful served with our Flax Tomato Crackers (see next page) and fresh vegetables.

Patty James Cooking School and Nutrition Centre for Grail Springs

Flax Tomato Crackers

You will need a food dehydrator for this recipe.

2 cups (500 ml) flax seeds
2 cups (500 ml) sun-dried tomato halves
1 chipotle pepper, dried, de-stemmed, seeds removed
3 garlic cloves
1 1/2 tablespoons (22.5 ml) dried basil
1 1/2 teaspoons (7.5 ml) dried oregano
1 1/2 teaspoons (7.5 ml) dried parsley
1 1/2 teaspoons (7.5 ml) Himalayan salt

- Soak flax seeds in 4 cups (1 L) of water for 20 minutes. The flax seeds should soak up all the water.
- Soak sun-dried tomatoes and chipotle pepper in 2 cups water until soft (about 20 minutes).
- Drain, reserving the soaking liquid for another use.
- Puree the tomatoes and pepper and garlic in a blender or food processor until smooth.
- Wash blender/processor and pulse flax seeds in 3 different batches until the seeds are broken.
- In a large bowl add the ground flax sees, the tomato, and garlic mixture and the seasonings. Stir well.
- Spread the mixture on a non-stick baking sheet until thin, using a spatula or your wet fingers.
- Dehydrate at 108F for approximately 16 hours. Turn over and dry another 2–4 hours until crispy.
- Store in an airtight container.

15 Servings
Serving ideas: Great served with Sprouted Garbanzo Hummus (see page 154) or Lime-scented Spinach Spread (see page 153).

Patty James Cooking School and Nutrition Centre for Grail Springs

Yogurt Cheese

4 cups (1 L) plain yogurt
2 cloves garlic, minced
2 tablespoons (30 ml) sun-dried tomato halves,
reconstituted in water. (Save water for another use.)
3 tablespoons (45 ml) Greek olives, sliced
1/2 teaspoon (2.5 ml) Himalayan salt

- Line a colander with cheesecloth and place it over
  a bowl.
- Pour the yogurt into the cheesecloth-lined colander.
  Bring up the sides of the cheesecloth and put a small
  bowl on top to act as a weight.
- Place in the refrigerator until all the liquid has drained
  into the bowl, about 24 hours. Be sure to pour out the
  liquid occasionally.
- When the "cheese" is ready, add the remaining
  ingredients and serve with your favourite crackers or as
  a vegetable dip.

Serves 10

Serving ideas: Alter at will. Add fresh dill in the summer and serve
with cold-poached salmon.

Patty James Cooking School and Nutrition Centre for Grail Springs

Red Lentil Dahl

1 cup (250 ml) red lentils
1 onion, diced
1 carrot, diced
1 stalk celery, diced
2 cloves garlic, minced
1 teaspoon (5 ml) ground cumin
1/2 teaspoon (2.5 ml) cinnamon
3 cups (750 ml) water or vegetable broth
Sea salt to taste

- Rinse red lentils well in cool water.
- Sweat vegetables until they start to get tender, add the spices and toast until you can smell them.
- Add the rinsed lentils and stir.
- Once everything is coated, add the water and simmer on very low for about an hour or until the lentils have cooked down to a puree, adding more liquid if needed.
- Season with salt to taste

Serves 4

Gomashio

2 teaspoons (10 ml) coarse Himalayan salt
5 teaspoons (25 ml) sesame seeds

- Toast the salt and sesame seeds, stirring frequently until aromatic.
- Allow them to cool and grind them in a clean coffee grinder. (Then clean coffee grinder!)

Serving ideas: Sprinkle on anything!

Patty James Cooking School and Nutrition Centre for Grail Springs

Arugula Pesto

1 cup (250 ml) arugula leaves
1 cup (250 ml) Italian parsley
2 cloves garlic
1/2 cup (125 ml) olive oil
1/4 cup (50 ml) Romano cheese
1 teaspoon (5 ml) Himalayan salt
1/2 teaspoon (2.5 ml) lemon juice, freshly squeezed

- Place all ingredients in a blender or food processor and puree.

Serves 8

Serving ideas: Wonderful served on grilled vegetables or grilled fish, as well as pasta. Can be refrigerated for a few days.

Patty James Cooking School and Nutrition Centre for Grail Springs

Cilantro Pesto

1 bunch cilantro, washed and dried
2 cloves garlic
1/4 cup (50 ml) pine nuts
1 tablespoon (15 ml) feta cheese
1/4 cup (50 ml) flax, hemp or olive oil
Sea salt and pepper

- Blend all ingredients together in a food processor or blender until smooth.
- If using hemp or flax oil, do not heat, just toss with warm vegetables or pasta.

Lime Scented Spinach Spread

10 oz (300 g) frozen spinach, thawed, drained and
   squeezed dry
2/3 cup (150 ml) scallions, chopped
1/2 package tofu, silken
1/4 cup (50 ml) lime juice
1 teaspoon (5 ml) lime zest
1 1/2 teaspoon (7.5 ml) Dijon mustard
1 teaspoon raw sugar
1/2 teaspoon Himalayan salt
1/2 teaspoon fresh ground pepper

- Combine spinach and scallions in food processor and
  pulse for about 30 seconds until blended.
- Add silken tofu, lime juice and zest, Dijon, sugar, salt
  and pepper to taste.
- Process until smooth.

Yield: 1 1/2 cups

Serving ideas: Garnish with lime zest. Serve with crackers, bread
or vegetables.

Patty James Cooking School and Nutrition Centre for Grail Springs

Sprouted Garbanzo Hummus

You will need a seed sprouter for this recipe.

1 cup (250 ml) garbanzo beans, sprouted

1 tablespoon (15 ml) tahini

1 tablespoon (15 ml) lemon juice

1 teaspoon (5 ml) olive oil

1 clove garlic

1/2 teaspoon (2.5 ml) Himalayan salt

1/2 teaspoon (2.5 ml) fresh ground pepper

- Soak the garbanzo beans in cold water over night.
- In the morning drain the beans and place in a sprouter until they begin to open (about 3–4 days), rinsing twice a day.
- Blend all ingredients in a blender until smooth.

Yields: 1 cup of dip

Serving ideas: Great on Flax Tomato Crackers (see page 147).

Patty James Cooking School and Nutrition Centre for Grail Springs

Nutmeg Sauce

3/4 cup (175 ml) raw sugar

2 tablespoons (30 ml) whole wheat flour

1 teaspoon (5 ml) nutmeg, freshly ground

1 cup (250 ml) boiling water

1 tablespoon (15 ml) unsalted butter

1 teaspoon (5 ml) vanilla

- In a small saucepan combine sugar, flour, and nutmeg. Gradually add water.
- Cook, stirring until thickened. Blend in butter and vanilla.

Yield: 1 1/2 cups

Serving Ideas: Serve warm over waffles, pancakes, crepes, or ice cream.

Patty James Cooking School and Nutrition Centre for Grail Springs

Braised Artichokes and Peas

2 large artichokes
1/2 lemon
2 tablespoons (30 ml) olive oil
1 1/2 teaspoons (7.5 ml) garlic, minced
3 tablespoons (45 ml) shallots, chopped
1/3 cup (75 ml)
2 pounds (910 g) fresh peas
2 tablespoons (30 ml) parsley, chopped
Dash Himalayan salt

- Trim the artichokes of all their tough parts. As you work, rub the cut artichoke with the lemon to keep it from turning dark.
- Cut artichoke lengthwise into 4 equal sections. Remove the soft curling leaves with prickly tips, and cut away the fuzzy choke. Detach the stems, and squeeze lemon over all the cut parts.
- Use an enamelled cast iron pot just large enough to accommodate all of the ingredients.
- Sauté chopped shallots in olive oil, on medium-high. Cook and stir the shallots until they very pale gold, then add the garlic. Cook the garlic until it becomes a light gold, then put in the artichoke wedges and 1/3 cup water. Adjust the heat to cook at a steady simmer; covered tightly.
- Shell the fresh peas and put aside.
- When the artichokes have cooked for about 10 minutes, add the shelled peas, parsley, and salt to taste and add more water if necessary. Stir the peas to coat them well.

- Cover tightly again, and continue cooking until the artichokes feel tender at their thickest point when prodded with a fork.
- Taste and correct for salt.

Serves 4

Serving ideas: Wonderful served with baked salmon and brown basmati rice. You may drizzle the salmon with just a little lemon butter before serving.

Patty James Cooking School and Nutrition Centre for Grail Springs

Spring Rolls with Spicy Almond Sauce

1 package of rice paper wrappers

1 carrot

1 stalk celery

1 green pepper

1 red pepper

1 cup (250 ml) cooked rice cellophane noodles

Marinade

1 tablespoon (15 ml) hemp seeds

1 tablespoon (15 ml) rice vinegar

1/2 teaspoon (2.5 ml) sesame oil

1/2 teaspoon (2.5 ml) Himalayan salt

Juice of one lime

- Thinly slice all the vegetables and set aside.
- Mix the marinade ingredients and pour over the vegetables.
- Marinate for 3–4 hours.
- Chop the cooked rice noodles into bite-size lengths and add to the vegetables.
- Soak each rice paper wrappers in water for 30 seconds and then drain on a towel.
- Put a 1/4 cup (50 ml) of the vegetable mixture on the edge of the rice paper and roll or wrap the rice paper around it.

For the Sauce

    2 tablespoons (30 ml) almond butter

    1 teaspoon (5 ml) wheat free soy sauce

    1/4 teaspoon (0.625 ml) sambal hot sauce

    1 tablespoon (15 ml) water

- Mix all ingredients together and use for a dipping sauce.

Yield: 10–12 spring rolls

Quinoa Fennel Pilaf

1 cup (250 ml) quinoa

1/2 small onion, finely chopped

1 rib celery, diced

1 carrot, diced

1 fennel bulb, trimmed, cored and diced

1 tablespoon (15 ml) unsalted butter

1 tablespoon (15 ml) olive oil

1 3/4 cups (425 ml) vegetable stock

- Rinse quinoa in a fine sieve.
- Sauté onion, celery, carrot and fennel in butter in a 3-quart (3 L) heavy saucepan over medium heat, stirring occasionally, until onion is softened, 7–8 minutes.
- Add quinoa and sauté over medium-high heat, stirring 2–3 minutes. Add stock and salt to taste.
- Cover and cook over low heat until quinoa is tender and liquid is absorbed (approx 12–15 minutes).

Serves 6

Serving ideas: Serve with Pecan Crusted Chicken (see page 138) and steamed seasonal vegetables.

Patty James Cooking School and Nutrition Centre for Grail Springs

Cashew Cream Sauce

This sauce can be made sweet or savoury – one can be used as a dessert topping while the other can be used as a salad dressing or a veggie dip.

Cashew Cream Sweet

    3 cups (750 ml) cashews

    1 cup (250 ml) water

    1$1/2$ teaspoons (7.5 ml) vanilla

    7 tablespoons (105 ml) maple syrup

Cashew Cream Savoury

    3 cups (750 ml) cashews

    1 cup (250 ml) water

    1$1/2$ teaspoon (7.5 ml) Dijon mustard

    1 tablespoon (15 ml) capers or olive, chopped

- For both recipes, grind cashews in food processor while pouring in water in a slow stream.
- Stir in remaining ingredients

Patty James Cooking School and Nutrition Centre for Grail Springs

Tahini-Garlic Sauce

1 tbsp tahini
1 large clove of garlic
splash of apple cider vinegar
splash of maple syrup
3/4 cup spring water

- Blend all ingredients with a hand blender, adding water just a bit at a time to get your desired consistency. Adjust flavours to your liking.

Dancing Beans Salsa

If you're roasting corn on the barbecue, save an ear for this recipe. The slightly charred flavour and blackened color add great earthiness to this summer salsa with substance.

This will make a big bowl for the whole family

1 cup organic black beans, soaked overnight and cooked
   (or 1 can of organic black beans, drained)
1 large or 2 medium ripe organic heirloom tomatoes, diced
1 small red onion, diced finely
1 small ripe mango, diced
1 red pepper, diced
1 ear of organic summer corn, roasted
1 ripe avocado, diced
fresh cilantro, chopped for garnish
1 clove of garlic, minced (I always use more)
juice of 1 lemon or lime
$1/2$ tsp cumin (or a little more to taste)
$1/2$ tsp chili powder (or more to taste)
1 tsp Himalayan sea salt

- Drain the beans and combine all ingredients in a large stainless steel bowl. Taste and adjust seasoning to your liking. Serve atop whole grain toasties, bruschetta-style, as a side to any salad, in a quesadilla with soy cheese, or simply with good quality organic corn chips.

Mango Chutney

1 ripe mango, finely diced
1 inch piece of fresh ginger, minced
1/2 tsp crushed chili flakes
1 lime, juiced
1 green onion, chopped finely

• Combine all ingredients and serve at room temperature.

Asparagus Spears & Cashew "Cream"

1 bunch spring asparagus, stems snipped

1 cup of raw cashews

1/2 lemon

pinch Himalayan sea salt

fresh pepper

- Place asparagus in an inch of water in a frying pan on high. Bring to a boil and cook for 1 minute.
- Meantime, in a powerful blender, mix cashews with juice from half a juicy lemon, a splash of water and a pinch of sea salt. Blend on high until creamy and smooth. Adjust consistency with a little more water if you need it. You should be able to pour the "cream" from the blender, but it should still be rich and thick.
- Take asparagus from the stove and plate. Pour cashew "cream" over the asparagus and grind fresh pepper over the whole dish. Serve as a delightful vegan side to any meal.

Serves 2–4

Sunflower Seed Pate

1 cup of organic sunflower seeds, soaked overnight

1 carrot

1 celery stalk

4 rounds of a medium eggplant

1/4 onion

3 cloves of garlic

1 tablespoon tahini

splash of tamari

1/2 teaspoon each, parsley, rosemary, oregano, basil

a pinch of thyme and sage

1 teaspoon Himalayan sea salt

1/2 cup of nutritional yeast

- Rinse and drain sunflower seeds.
- Brush a little olive oil on rounds of eggplant and roast in the oven at 400 until soft.
- Blend all ingredients in a cuisinart or blender until they're well blended – not a puree, you want to leave a few chunks, but everything should stick together. If it seems a bit dry, add a splash of water.
- Taste and adjust seasoning to your liking – a bit more tamari, some more nutritional yeast, a pinch more sage…
- Put in a baking vessel of some sort, like a small glass casserole pan or a small loaf pan. Muffin tins will also work for making little baby pates.
- Bake at 300 for about 40 minutes or until lightly browned on top.

Serves 6–8

Serve with raw celery, carrots, radishes, tomatoes and greens. Or spread warm on rice cakes and serve with greens and raw veggies.

Raw Nut "Cream"

1/2 cup raw organic almonds, soaked overnight
1/2 cup raw organic cashews, soaked overnight
1/4 cup raw organic pine nuts, soaked overnight
1 lemon, juiced
Himalayan sea salt to taste
Spring water

- Drain, then combine soaked almonds, cashews and pine
  nuts in a powerful blender. Add a splash of water and the
  juice of a whole lemon and blend. Keep adding water until
  you achieve your desired creamy consistency. Add a pinch
  of sea salt and blend again, making sure all the nuts are
  blended.

"Angry-Style" Ancient Grain

Spelt is an ancient grain related to wheat. It contains more protein, and is easier to digest than wheat. Most people who are allergic to wheat can tolerate spelt, and therefore a lot of baked goods and pastas are now made with spelt flour.

I enjoy the whole, unprocessed grain for its sweet, deeply nutty flavour and chewy consistency. This recipe uses sprouted spelt instead of pasta as the carrier of a wonderful "angry-style" spicy tomato sauce.

2 cups of whole organic spelt, soaked for 24 hours in
   spring water

6 or 7 cloves of garlic, minced

1 tbsp olive oil

1 tsp sambal oelek or dried red chilis

1 shallot, finely diced

1/2 red onion, finely diced

3 large ripe organic tomatoes, diced

1 tsp Himalayan sea salt

1 sprig each, fresh parsley, basil, rosemary

1/4 cup pine nuts, toasted

- Rinse and soak whole spelt for at least 24 hours in spring water, rinsing a couple of times throughout the 24-hour period.
- In a cast iron pan, sautee garlic in olive oil on medium heat. Add chilis, shallot and red onion. Stir until soft.
- Drain and add the whole spelt, stirring to mix with the garlic and onion.

- Add diced tomatoes and Himalayan sea salt to the pan and stir until the ingredients are well blended. Simmer for 10 minutes.
- Chop parsley and basil and add to sauce just before serving.
- Taste and adjust seasoning. Perhaps you like it a bit spicier…add more chilis or a pinch of cayenne pepper.
- Garnish with a sprig of rosemary and top with toasted pine nuts. Serve with a side of fresh organic greens drizzled with hemp or flax seed oil and apple cider vinegar.

Serves 2–4

Desserts

Dr. Haas' Banana Nice Cream

You must use a Champion Juicer with the hook-up that pushes out everything in order to make this recipe.

- Peel and freeze one bunch of bananas
- Push each whole banana through the juicer. They will come out creamy banana nice cream.
- You may sprinkle carob, raw chocolate, hemp, walnuts, almonds, pecans or berries for variation.

Another alternative: For a frozen yogurt delight, put the creamy banana nice cream in blender, add yogurt, honey, maple syrup or cinnamon to taste. Put the mixture into freezer-safe cups and into the freezer.

Yummm!

Chocolate Torte

Filling

1 package silken tofu

3/4 cup (175 ml) rice milk

1/2 cup (125 ml) packed pitted dates

1/2 cup (125 ml) organic cocoa powder

2 tablespoons (30 ml) melted coconut oil

1 teaspoon (5 ml) pure vanilla

1/4 tsp (1.25 ml) orange zest

Crust

1/2 cup (125 ml) unsweetened flaked coconut

1/4 cup (50 ml) pitted dates

1/2 cup (125 ml) ground raw almonds

3/4 cup (175 ml) buckwheat flour

Pinch Himalayan Salt

Pinch cardamom

Pinch cinnamon

2 tablespoons (30 ml) coconut oil

- For the crust, blend the almonds and dates in a food processor.
- Remove to a large bowl and add the rest of the ingredients.
- Knead until it forms a ball.
- Press into a 9-inch round pan or pie plate and chill.
- For the filling blend all ingredients in a processor until smooth and pour into your chilled crust.
- Chill until firm and serve.

Serves 8

Coconut Cream Pie

Crust

    1 cup (250 ml) raw cashews

    1/2 cup (125 ml) raw almonds

    1 egg

    2 tablespoons (30 ml) honey

    1/2 cup (125 ml) spelt flour

    1/4 cup (50 ml) rice milk

    Pinch sea salt

Filling

    3 eggs

    2 tablespoons (30 ml) honey

    2 cups (500 ml) coconut milk

    2 teaspoons (10 ml) pure vanilla

- To make the crust, blend all ingredients in a food processor until it forms a ball. Press into a 9-inch pan and set aside to chill.
- To make the filling, combine the eggs and honey and whisk together.
- Heat the coconut milk until scalded and whisk gradually into the egg mixture.
- Stir in the vanilla.
- Pour into chilled crust and bake at 350F (180C) for approximately 20–25 minutes or until custard is set.

Serves 8

Gingerbread

1 tablespoon (15 ml) maple syrup

3/4 cup (175 ml) packed pitted dates

1/3 cup (75 ml) coconut oil

1 1/2 cups (375 ml) milk (soy, almond, rice)

1 1/2 cups (375 ml) spelt flour

2/3 cup (150 ml) brown rice flour

1/4 teaspoon (1.25 ml) baking soda

1 1/2 teaspoon (7.5 ml) baking powder

1 tablespoon (15 ml) cinnamon

1 tablespoon (15 ml) fresh ginger, grated

2 eggs

- Blend maple syrup, dates, oil and milk together in a blender or food porcessor until smooth and set aside.
- Sift together dry ingredients in a large bowl.
- Form a well in the centre of dry ingredients and pour in wet mixture.
- Whisk eggs and add to bowl.
- Pour into greased 9 x 9-inch square pan.
- Bake at 375F (190C) for 30 minutes or until cake tester comes out clean.

To serve 8–10

Bean Brownie

3/4 cup (185 ml) adzuki beans

1/2 cup (125 ml) maple syrup

2/3 cup (150 ml) vegetable oil

3/4 cup (175 ml) organic cocoa

1 1/2 teaspoon (7.5 ml) sea salt

1 1/2 teaspoon (7.5 ml) pure vanilla

3/4 cup (185 ml) spelt flour

6 eggs

- Adzuki beans do not need to be soaked so they can be cooked in water until tender, about 45–50 minutes.
- Puree the beans with everything but the flour and eggs.
- Mix the puree and the flour together.
- In a separate bowl, whisk the eggs then fold them into the batter.
- Pour into a 9 x 9-inch pan and bake at 350F (180C) for 20–30 minutes.

Serves 6–8

Spiced Cashew Ice Cream

1 cup (250 ml) raw unsalted cashews

1 cup (250 ml) pure water, plus more for soaking

1 cup (250 ml) almond milk

1/4 cup (50 ml) packed pitted dates

1 teaspoon (5 ml) pure vanilla extract

1 teaspoon (5 ml) cardamom

1/2 teaspoon (2.5 ml) cinnamon

1/2 teaspoon (2.5 ml) fresh grated nutmeg

1/8 teaspoon (0.625 ml) Himalayan salt

- Soak cashews in water for at least 2 hours.
- Discard soaking water.
- Add all ingredients to a blender and blend on high until smooth. For added smoothness strain through a mesh strainer after blending.
- Chill in fridge or freezer for half-an-hour, then freeze in an ice cream maker until set. Serve right away or store in the freezer.

Yield: 4 cups (1 L)

Raw Carrot Cake

1 large carrot, grated finely

1 cup organic raisins, soaked in spring water then
    chopped finely

2 cups whole walnuts, chopped finely

1/2 cup organic coconut

1 lg tbsp tahini

quarter cup maple syrup

1 tsp vanilla

pinch each cinnamon, nutmeg, clove

1 tsp coconut oil for pan

- Mix all ingredients in a large bowl, then press firmly into a small round pan oiled lightly with coconut oil. Let sit for at least an hour before serving.

Vegan "Cream Cheese" Icing

1 cup cashews

juice from 1 lemon

splash water

quarter cup maple syrup

tsp vanilla

- Blend on high to create smooth, creamy, thick consistency, then spread over cake.

Chef's tips: Try blending first just with lemon juice and maple syrup, then add a little splash of water as you need more liquid. A powerful Vita-Mix on high speed will help to make a silky creamy texture. mmm.

Remember, there's no flour holding the cake together. Extracting the carrot cake in a nice wedge requires an angel's touch.

Truffles for Angels

Revered the world over for its sweet taste and creamy texture, chocolate is considered by many to be an aphrodisiac — and a perfect dessert or gift for loved ones on Valentine's Day or any other special day.

Ancient Aztec Indians believed that eating the fruit from the cacao tree brought wisdom and power. The legend, still alive today, if you ask any chocolate lover, was that cacao seeds had been brought from Paradise.

Dark chocolate has been shown in studies to help prevent heart disease and some cancers, and is known to enhance moods by boosting the brain chemical serotonin, much in the way that modern anti-depressant drugs work.

These dairy-free chocolate truffles will cure what ails you — and bring you and your guests rapturous delight!

1 1/2 cups raw cashews

3 dozen organic dates

1/2 an organic lemon

1/2 tsp vanilla extract

Half a pound of high quality organic fair trade dark chocolate.

   (Or 1 package of dark chocolate vegan baking chips.)

- Place dates in a small saucepan and add enough spring water to cover bottom of pan. Bring to a boil and simmer while stirring until dates soften and a thick "date jam" is formed.
- Turn off heat and allow to cool.
- In a powerful blender or cuisinart, blend cashews, juice of lemon, dates and vanilla extract.
- Place in a bowl in the freezer and allow to harden for an hour or overnight.

- In a double boiler, melt the dark chocolate to liquid. Keep the heat on minimum once it's melted, and work quickly.
- Using a melon-baller or a small round spoon, scoop out the cashew-date mixture and drop into a larger round spoon. Ladle melted chocolate over the ball, covering it entirely. Set truffle on a cookie sheet lined with parchment paper and dusted with organic cocoa powder. (For Valentine's Day, use a heart-shaped candy mould.)
- When you're finished, there should be about 3 dozen Truffles for Angels. Put the cookie sheet in the fridge to allow the chocolate to set. Once they've set, you can take them out and store them in a cool place.
- Arrange beautifully on a plate and sprinkle with organic cocoa powder.

Yields 3 dozen

chapter 5
Purify Thyself!

Now that we've covered the food portion of your holistic detox plan, it's time to take care of the rest of you. After choosing to embark on a cleanse, keep in mind that adding the following regimens wherever possible will optimize your detox experience. All of the following are practices that we have integrated into our programs at Grail Springs.

Prepare the Skin
Exfoliation and Dry Brushing

Preparing the skin is essential. Salt scrubs or dry brushes are excellent ways to wake up the body and prepare your skin to eliminate toxins, which is one of its most important functions. The skin is responsible for eliminating one third of the body's waste each day — the total waste a body expels can amount to one pound per day. While you are dry brushing the skin you are also providing a gentle massage to the organs. Purchase a simple dry brush, with soft natural bristles or a loofa. You can even use a rolled up face cloth if you can't find a brush. Stand in the shower or tub with the water off. Beginning with your feet, start to rub your skin in circular motions using firm but gentle pressure. Always work towards the direction of the heart. Avoid the face and irritated skin. This whole process should only take you five minutes and can be done prior to showering each morning.

Other benefits to incorporating skin brushing into your daily regime:
1. Tightens the skin and prevents premature aging
2. Tones the muscles
3. Cleanses the lymphatic system
4. Removes cellulite
5. Improves circulation
6. Stimulates digestion
7. Improves the function of the nervous system

The Alchemist's Bath
Toxins Out – Minerals In!

Mother Earth's Magic Potions

Minerals play a huge role in our body's ability to function and stay healthy. Ninety-five per cent of our body's functions, like the simple task of just thinking, are dependant on minerals being present. Supplementing the body's mineral intake through natural products from the earth is one very potent way to acquire the necessary minerals we need to stay energized.

End each day of your detox program with a detox bath. I suggest using Himalayan bath salts, Austrian moor mud or organic seaweed powders. These gifts from Mother Earth will not only help to draw out the toxins but what they offer up in the way of minerals is simply amazing. These are all my personal favorites, each providing extraordinary results and a slightly different experience.

Transform your bathroom into a wellness and water sanctuary

Set the mood with aromatherapy candles, soft lighting and relaxing instrumental music. This should be a restful and much anticipated experience each night. It's an excellent opportunity for you to wind down with some quiet meditation and practice some deep, smooth breathing techniques. Open a window and let in some fresh air, which will also help create a bit of a steam bath. Enjoy a cup of decaffeinated tea like mint or chamomile. Soak for 20 to 30 minutes. Place a nice cold, wet facecloth over your forehead if you find yourself experiencing a really good sweat.

[
All Medicine is in the Earth
– Paracelsus
]

Add ons...

I always take the opportunity to add a hair and scalp oil treatment and a mud or seaweed mask to my routine. The steam from the bath helps to activate these clarifying masks that detox the skin and reduce puffy eyes or swelling. Tibetan hair oil is one of the best products I have found on the market. Made from apricot kernels this oil helps with premature greying and to my unexpected astonishment, helped with new hair growth. I simply pin my hair up and place a towel on my pillow for the night and rinse out in the morning with Austrian moor mud shampoo and conditioner. The combination makes for very healthy hair and a healthy scalp which we often forget needs just as much attention.

When you are finished with your bath, do not rub your skin dry, simply pat or air dry naturally. Do not apply any lotions following your bath, as the elements will continue to process for several hours and through the night. Wear unrestricted cotton pyjamas and use cotton linens on your bed. Avoid synthetics. Curl up with an inspirational book and enjoy a restful, peaceful sleep. This is a perfect way to end each day of your detox program. These detox baths will alkalize your body, act as a gentle detox and decrease any discomfort you might have from inflammation or skin irritations. You will see a noticeable difference in the texture of your skin.

New Moon = Detox = toxins out
Full Moon = Replenishment = minerals in

During the full moon the body will more readily absorb minerals and heal. You can work with these natural rhythms of the moon to optimize which results you want.

As mentioned previously, if you can choose a week when the moon is in a new phase, you will optimize your detox results. The rhythm of a new moon supports weight loss and detoxification.

Have a thermometer on hand to gauge the temperature of the water. Water in a detox bath should be approximately 98.6F. (This is the temperature of the amniotic fluid in the womb.)

Austrian Moor Mud

With over 1,000 herbs and 100 organic compounds plus a host of trace elements, vitamins, phtyo-hormones, and essential oils, mud from Austria's famous Moor is one of nature's most potent healing compounds. The remarkable rejuvenating effects of the Moor have been known since at least 800 B.C. Recent excavations have uncovered ancient Celtic and Roman baths fully preserved in the Moors of Austria. Ancient chronicles from the area refer to its "mysterious healing properties," and observations from local people reveal the positive effect on injured animals, and people who sought out, bathed in, and drank from the Moor.

In the sixteenth century, Paracelsus, a famous physician and alchemist, sent his patients to bathe in the Moor baths based on his influential theory of the *quinta essentia vitae* on the five main bio-chemical properties of the Moor. He believed he had discovered in the Moor the ultimate remedy or "Elixir of Life." The moor was formed at the end of the Ice Age nearly 30,000 years ago when myriad species of herbs, plants, and flowers were submerged under a lake formed by melting glacial waters. Protected from the ravages of oxygen, the herbs gradually assimilated into a rich black magma with all of their medicinal components intact. The result is a compound with quite spectacular revitalizing properties.

Himalayan Salt

Over 70% of our planet is covered with ocean. This water and salt solution embodies the essential energy for the creation of life. We have come to understand through the science of biophysics that water and salt combined have holistic qualities that can help us to maintain our health and prevent many ailments. The mix of the two is called "sole" from the Latin word for sun, "sol."

[
"...all of us have in our veins the exact
same percentage of salt in our blood that
exists in the ocean. We have salt in our
blood, in our sweat, in our tears. We are
tied to the ocean."
]

– John F. Kennedy

Mythologically it means "liquid sunlight," the materialization of the sun's energy. This can also make for a great meditation when in the bath – imagine yourself bathing in liquid sunlight. The beauty of the pink salt that is mined from the Himalayas is that it is 100% pure and contains 84 natural elements found in and needed by the body, which can be easily metabolized. This crystal salt is full of life. When bathing on a new moon cycle, it will draw toxins out of the body. A bath in "sole" water can have the same affect as a three-day fast. When bathing on the full moon cycle it will have a replenishing effect.

Organic Seaweed

Seaweed powder added to a bath can have a wonderful detoxifying effect. Seaweed can delay the aging process because of the ease with which it can penetrate the skin with good nutrients, anti-oxidants, minerals, and trace elements. Considering that the minerals and trace elements in ocean water are proportional to that of human blood plasma, seaweed has proven valuable in complementary therapies. Whether applied topically or taken internally, kelp and seaweed aid in moisture retention and contain amino acids to help firm and renew skin tissue. Seaweed can improve lymph and blood circulation, stimulate cellular metabolism, increase fluidity of cellular membranes and fight against inflammation. One of the finest and purest sources of seaweed today is harvested from the coast of Vancouver Island in British

Columbia; this is the only seaweed we choose to utilize at Grail Springs. Scientists report that this particular seaweed is rich in vitamins A1, B1, B2, B6, B12, folic acid, and niacin, with significant amounts of vitamins C, E, and K. It also supplies us with an excellent source of over 60 minerals, especially potassium, calcium, iodine, magnesium, phosphorus, iron, zinc, and manganese. Seaweed is simply a treasure trove of nutritional concentrates.

Sleeping for Health & Wellbeing

Sleep is a natural state of rest for all life forms and necessary for survival. According to Ayurvedic practices, the best cycle for humans to sleep is from 10:00 PM to 6:00 AM when sleep comes most easily. Morning is a natural detox time when our body wants to eliminate waste. From 10:00 AM to 2:00 PM our body is at its highest metabolic rate so that is a good time to have our main meal. Humans are diurnal creatures, meaning that we do best rising with the sun and resting after sundown.

The National Sleep Foundation states that adults need eight to nine hours of sleep to maintain optimum levels of alertness, memory, and overall health, though many would claim they need less, around six to eight hours. Listen to your body and your needs, but know that sleep is a time for regeneration. Losing sleep can take its toll on your body and psyche if it becomes a pattern. Anyone who has experienced staying up late to study for exams or nursed a sick child or suffered anxiety-related insomnia, knows what sleep deprivation can do to one's state of mind. We can get very irritable and find it difficult to focus or concentrate and be prone to accidents. It is important to speak to your naturopath if this has become an ongoing problem. Many people have bad memories associated with bedtime such as family arguments, bedwetting, nightmares, and fear of the dark. At one point in my life I shuddered at the thought of night time. A workaholic at the time, I used to think to myself, "Let's just get this sleep thing over with so I can get back to work." I thought it a complete waste of time and resisted it, which never allowed for a full and restful night's sleep and added to my ongoing health problem. When we are grieving or worried it seems the daylight makes it easier to bear while the night seems almost unbearable. There can be all kind of psychological reasons for people to resist sleep.

Tips for creating better sleep patterns

- Make your bedroom a restful sanctuary,
  your favourite place on earth
- Keep your bedroom tidy and uncluttered
- Keep your bedroom an electronics-free zone
- Rest and rise at the same time each day,
  creating a pattern for your body to follow
- Exercise in the morning, rather than in the evening,
  if you can
- Avoid eating after 7:00 PM
- Keep your bedroom at a cool and comfortable
  temperature
- Invest in good quality cotton linens,
  orthopaedic pillows and mattress
- Pay attention to the lighting; keep it soft
  and unobtrusive

Embracing relaxation and using all the tools at your disposal such as meditation to reduce stress levels, yoga, getting regular massages, taking evening detox baths, all of these integrated into your life plan will eventually induce a better sleep pattern. Embrace sleep wholeheartedly as a time for health restoration and for your mental wellbeing. Mornings don't have to be a race to the coffee maker but rather an optimum time for silent meditation, breath work, gratitude invocation, and creative visioning.

The Breath of Life

Take a full deep breath in through your nose slowly, filling up with air right down to the bottom of your stomach. Exhale through your mouth. Take another. And another. Did you know you've just charged your entire body, mind, and spirit with sunlight! Oxygen carries the life-giving energy force of the sun. You might have even felt a little tingling sensation towards the tips of your toes. Try it again and see if you can feel it this time.

Breath work has to be the most powerful yet underrated technique for transforming health and wellbeing. Though the knowledge is ancient, originating from yoga schools of thought as "Pranayama," it is a rarely understood essential element that directly affects our state of health. Our breathing is probably the most disconnected and most neglected element of our health in North America. Perhaps it is just too easy and seems so obvious. Maybe that is why it has been overlooked.

There is a right way to breathe and a wrong way. Deep breathing alkalizes the body, while short breathing acidifies the body which does not make for a happy body. By limiting our breathing to the upper part of the chest only, we are also signaling our nervous system to pump up our adrenals which can cause great stress, sometimes to dangerous levels. When our nervous system is not properly regulated our heart has to pump that much faster while other normal functions of the body also start to react in a negative way. Simply said, a lack of oxygen exhausts us, can cause "burn out" and ultimately premature death. You only have to look at how quickly we die from lack of oxygen. There is no other essential element without which even for just a few minutes we can not live.

Deep breathing alkalizes the body, while short breathing acidifies the body!

Pranayama speaks to the use of right control of "energy" through the process of inhalation and exhalation. Prana means "energy" not "breath" as some might think. The method refers to the right use of breathing so that we can optimize our prana (energy). Prana is the life force behind all living organisms. Every living organism breathes in and exhales out. There exists a natural ebb and flow of energy in every living being. This is powered by prana itself!

We can control our energy by controlling our breath. It is not that we want to focus our attention to the physical breathing alone, what we want to understand here is how to use breathing to feed our "prana," our vital energy, which then flows to our nervous system and our cellular structure. Every cell, organ, nerve, muscle in our body is waiting to be replenished with a blast of oxygen in order for it to function smoothly. Stop that flow we run into trouble.

So we want to be cognizant of the importance of maintaining a nice steady stream of healthy oxygen into our lungs in order to cleanse ourselves. When you are more conscious of breathing properly, keep in mind that you are fueling all of you – body, heart, mind, and spirit and cleansing everything at the same time. It is a very powerful feeling.

Oxygen feeds it all...

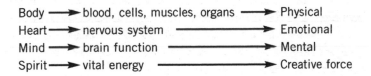

Body ⟶ blood, cells, muscles, organs ⟶ Physical
Heart ⟶ nervous system ⟶ Emotional
Mind ⟶ brain function ⟶ Mental
Spirit ⟶ vital energy ⟶ Creative force

Breath work could and should be recognized as "the next big thing" in complementary medicine. Dr. Andrew Weil, renowned author, speaker, proponent of complementary medicine, and director of Arizona University, prescribes breath work to many

Our prana, our life force, is what is drawing in the breath!

of his patients and teaches it to other medical doctors. He says in his book *Breathing: The Master Key to Self Healing* that prescribing breath work techniques to his patients has proven itself as one of the most effective solutions to resolving many health ailments such as insomnia, circulatory problems, digestion, anxiety, and much more.

In Qi Gong or yoga classes, students become aware of the importance of the breath and right posture. They learn to reduce and eliminate the unreleased tension of the mind and body. Ideally, flexibility can create in the body a state of balance that will enable the individual to move and breathe stress free. This lack of restriction can do wonders for digestion, healing, sleep deprivation, and many other health issues that people suffer from. Don't push it or overdo it. Right breathing will eventually come naturally.

Start integrating breath work into your life plan

No need to over think this. In fact it is not recommended. Simply start by removing obstacles that may be keeping you from getting enough fresh oxygen in your day:

- Make sure you are working in a oxygen-friendly environment with proper ventilation.
- Keep good posture.
- Be mindful about breathing in deep, full breaths, not shallow.
- Become smoke free. If you want to reach optimum health, we highly recommend that you seek the assistance of

a naturopathic doctor in order to address nicotine addiction.
- Get connected with the air you live and breathe in and start to relate to it as "energy" feeding your life force.
- Start and end your day with a couple of minutes of deep breathing.
- While you are sitting at your desk, driving in your car, or standing in a line up and the thought comes to mind, take a few deep breaths.
- Join a Yoga, Qi Gong or Tai Chi class in your area, all of which integrate breath work into their techniques.

Water
The Pillar of Life

Water is an extraordinary element and force of nature – one could write volumes about the research that has investigated its life-giving properties. Science still considers it a bit of an anomaly because it doesn't behave in a way that one expects. Thanks to recent documentaries like Al Gore's *An Inconvenient Truth*, governments and leaders of influence are starting to demand more specifically every day for the protection of our water and our environment. A fresh and healthy water supply cannot be taken for granted.

We know of the innate healing powers of spring water, said to be the best water in the world. Holy waters, some ancient and well known around the world such as Lourdes in France and the Chalice Well in England are all said to carry powerful properties for healing with thousands of documented cases.

["The solution to pollution is dilution."
– Dr. Elson Haas]

The spring waters that fill the lake here at Grail Springs play an essential role in the effectiveness of the therapies, the baths, the drinking water, and the overall success of the health programs. The water here is revered by many visitors for its unique properties and effectiveness. We do not contaminate the water with chlorine, but rather filter it through ultraviolet light and a sand filter and have it tested by an independent contractor every week.

The lake here at Grail Springs is alkaline based. It is fed by hundreds of vigorous springs, and comes bubbling up from the ancient granite bedrocks below the surface. We often refer to it affectionately as Grail's holy water, or liquid gold. The value of clean lake water cannot be taken for granted. We live in what is called the Canadian Precambrian Rock Shield, known to be the oldest exposed rock in the world, twisted and formed by the ice age, and estimated to be 1.6 billion years old. You can see the springs appear after the first cold winter night as the water patterns are captured on the surface. There is no public access on this lake and luckily there is a friendly acknowledgement amongst the neighbours to be respectful and protective of this rarity. The practice of using electric boat motors and human-powered boats like canoes, pedal boats and rowboats instead of high powered, fuel-injected boats is a responsible act in order to save small fresh water lakes, such as ours.

According to www.one.org, the campaign to make poverty history, "every 15 seconds a child dies from a disease associated with a lack of access to safe drinking water, adequate sanitation and hygiene."

Our body is an intelligent and brilliant being. It gives us all kinds of signals when it is not getting enough water. The body needs constant replenishment throughout the day in order to function with ease. Failing to take in enough water leads to dehydration. Dehydration leads to illness. Hydration gives life and heals.

Let water be a pillar in your life

- Hydrate thyself!
- Develop a new relationship and a new appreciation for water
- Honour and respect this energy life force: conserve and protect it
- Celebrate it

Saunas

Many cultures have recognized this process as a way of keeping young and vibrant, and use it regularly as an effective way to detox. One sitting for approximately 15 to 30 minutes can be the fastest way to remove toxins from our body as it comes out with the sweat from our pores. Repeated use of a sauna can help to restore the function of elimination which sometimes gets completely blocked.

Some people cannot tolerate saunas because of the heat; therefore the newest technology, infrared, is an excellent option. In an infrared sauna the air stays cool while only the inner core of the body heats up. Grail Springs has all three sauna types: steam, dry, and infrared. We particularly like the infrared dome because it burns calories, detoxifies, and reduces acid levels all at the same time. These new domes are practical, movable and can be purchased for home use.

Infrared light is absorbed by us from sunlight and is necessary to our vitality and wellbeing. Many of us don't get the proper dose of sunlight as we work inside buildings all day, and there are also real dangers to having too much sun. Infrared is capable of penetrating deep into the human body. It can gently elevate the body's temperature. When it does so, it helps to expand capillaries, which stimulates blood circulation. This increases the body's energy reserve and accelerates the metabolic exchange between blood and body tissue. Infrared can actually increase the body tissue's regenerative ability. Infrared's outstanding

[Remember to drink lots of water before and after a sauna or an infrared treatment.]

properties are gaining worldwide recognition and acclaim, and we are beginning to see it appear in a wide variety of applications. You will feel a great sense of well-being as the warmth of the infrared heat begins to penetrate. It improves oxygen levels, eliminates fat, chemicals, and toxins from the blood and other wastes as well. The treatment reduces the acidic levels of the body and helps to normalize your alkaline levels. And we are all for that here at Grail Springs!

Colon Health

This is a hot topic of conversation during any dinner hour at Grail Springs and nobody seems to mind a bit! It is quite astounding when you realize the connection between the state of the colon and the state of one's health. Colon cleansing is an optional part of the detox program, but something you might want to consider. Every organ, every gland and every cell is affected by the health condition of the large intestine, the colon.

Many historians trace the origins of colon cleansing back to the Egyptians who say their knowledge came directly from the gods themselves. Ancient papyrus scrolls reveal that the Egyptians believed even then that all disease began from diet, and in order to combat potential disease they cleared their colons once a month for three consecutive days using enemas. Today it is still considered a valuable technique to kick-start proper elimination and even reverse health conditions resulting from improper diet.

Health problems such as headaches, dermatitis, bad breath, fatigue, arthritis, stomach ailments, and heart disease have been linked to a congested colon. When colon health is compromised, the waste backs up, becomes toxic and is released through the bowel walls into the bloodstream. Cleaning the colon can lighten the toxic load. It is especially helpful if you can arrange to either see a recommended colon hydrotherapist in your area or consider two to three self-administered enemas during your cleansing process. You can purchase enema kits at your local pharmacy. Some of the immediate benefits you may see from a colon cleanse is clearer skin, clean breath, reduced bloating, and improved digestion and elimination.

Many diseases start in the colon. Set in motion a conscious regime that will create an upward cycle of rejuvenation internally to ensure optimum health and vitality for years to come. This along with a balanced acid/alkaline approach to your diet is the best form of preventative medicine.

It is especially important to follow a dos and don'ts list several days prior to doing a colon cleanse. Do not eat red meat, fried foods, or sweets. Do eat cooked grains, steamed vegetables, soups, vegetable juices, and sprouts. You can begin taking a daily fibre cleanse drink first thing in the morning using green super food powders and mix into a non citrus juice. It is also good to add flaxseed oil to your drink.

It is also recommended to take acidophilus five to seven days prior to a colon cleanse and chlorophyll during, to prepare and replenish the good intestinal bacteria to the colon which can get washed away during a cleanse.

Massage & Body Work

Of course none of us can ever receive enough hands-on massage or body work. Besides the obvious effects of willingly surrendering our control momentarily into a stranger's hands, and allowing ourselves to completely abandon our daily responsibilities and relax, the purpose of receiving a massage during a cleanse is to get the energy flowing and lymphatic fluids moving. This is imperative. Have massage therapy not just during a seasonal cleanse but routinely every couple of weeks, or at the least once a month.

Specifically during your cleanse it is recommended that you schedule yourself in for one massage around the second day and one on the last day. There are many traditional massage techniques available from traditional Swedish to more exotic techniques. Inform your massage therapists that you are in the middle of a detox cleanse and they will adapt their massage technique to suit. Have them also spend a little extra time massaging your lower abdominal region. Again, this will help with elimination which is important.

Body work that can optimize your detox experience:
- Swedish massage
- Deep tissue
- Rolfing
- Hot stone massage
- Chakra balancing
- Reflexology
- Hair and scalp massage
- Lymphatic drainage massage
- Lomi lomi
- Tai massage
- Shiatsu

Fitness & Movement

I know what you are thinking, "I knew this was coming!" How we think about something can determine the outcome, so before we even get started with introducing exercise into your detox regime, why don't we introduce a new perspective about exercise itself.

The Knighthood Training

My fitness trainer reminded me of the warrior mind-set. Ancient warriors such as medieval Knights or the Japanese Samurai from a mystical era in time, would conjure up thoughts of great power and strength. The ancient arts of the knighthoods or today's popular martial arts are disciplines of order, strategy, mindfulness, and respect. Teachings may vary between the disciplines, but ultimately it comes down to one universal truth. These master warriors both past and present learned to unlock the power of the mind to understand how to harness the energy within. Through the use of thought and breath, they could channel the flow of this energy in specific directions through the body and release it with great force. This was the skill to be had and what made the difference between living and dying.

The greater lesson, understood by the most revered, was the ultimate secret of these brotherhoods. "The greatest power of all comes from withholding power." In other words, these disciplines taught that force was not a right. It was only to be used to defend the innocent, and that being the aggressor was not the way of the masterful warrior. The way of the true warrior was through peace and self control.

Be Disciplined to Be Strong: That is the Point

Integrating exercise into a life plan is a discipline, not just physically, but mentally more than anything else. We all go through phases in our life during which we are excited about fitness for a moment and then lose steam and bail out for a while. Life takes us through many emotional and mental roller coaster rides and when this happens it affects our desire to move. We can become immobilized.

At this point in my personal life, now in my mid-forties, I have come to understand two things that have made the difference. It is these two things that motivate me every day to get up and get moving. It's changed my perspective about exercise.

First, when you feel disciplined and you feel strong, physically, at your core, you feel strong in every other way: emotionally, mentally, and spiritually. You feel invincible. It feels good to feel disciplined and strong.

Second, when you understand that you are an energetic being and start to connect with that inner force of unlimited power and potential, you gain a new respect for what you are really made up of. Self responsibility comes into play in the truest sense of the word. In other words I now feel happily obliged to take care of my body and keep the energy flowing.

My chiropractor, who is an excellent motivator, speaker, and coach, has a great love for running. He runs every morning rain or shine, and he once said to me that when he runs, it is a spiritual experience. I could sense and picture what he was saying in my mind but it was only recently when I started running every morning with my trainer that I really understood what he said. There is something very spiritual about it if you allow for that to come in to your life. It's just one more way to get "connected."

Fitness for Detox Cleansing
Fitness is ultimately what your body is counting on in order to keep things moving whether or not you are on a detox. In order to get the system in optimum working condition during a detox cleanse, the organs have to be massaged and the fluids kept moving.

Detox-friendly exercises:
- brisk walking
- Pilates
- yoga
- light skip rope jumping
- rebounders

 You can only be successful at something if you have an interest in it.

- trampolines

The key here is to find an exercise that gets you excited! Exercise is probably one of the easiest things to give up on quickly. It is often the one thing that gets sacrificed if we run out of time in our day. If you are just getting back on track for the first time in a long time, start with walking. Whatever you do, don't start something that you know is a strain or something you know you are not going to like. That won't serve you in the long run. How about starting off with a brisk walk to the park or around the block? Start small and just keep setting your sights on reaching new levels one step at a time. This is not a race; it's a life-long trek.

Find an instructor who inspires you and makes it interesting. I prefer to find someone who calls themselves a coach. An instructor instructs. A coach coaches. I like being coached. A coach will talk to you about their own personal experience. If your instructor or trainer doesn't get you excited, move on and find another. Sometimes it is not the fitness program that is boring, it's the instructor. There are some fantastic motivational trainers and coaches out there, each with their own unique perspective.

Yoga for instance, can be a way of life, not just an exercise. If you find an instructor who incorporates the yoga lifestyle perspective into their teaching you may adopt a new way of thinking and living as a result. Since being brought to North America yoga has taught millions of people how to transform stress and create calm in their life by incorporating meditation and breathing techniques, both important elements to achieving optimum health.

Once you've completed a detox program and are back on track and into a normal pattern, you can start to step up to a cardio program. A strong, healthy heart can be nurtured and cared for by you and you only. Be good to your own heart. Give it a good daily workout by doing some form of exercise.

Jumpin' Detox!

As well as being a motivational coach here at Grail Springs, I also have the great fortune of being a student, continuing to be taught by extraordinary and talented individuals who happen to come here as guests. On one particular day in 2006 it was 38-year-old Lucie B – a doctor turned fitness professional and Jump Rope Master Trainer. She was the 2005 U.S. National Jump Rope Champion, 2006/2007 National Bronze Medalist for speed and power, and 2007 Regional Jump Rope champion in freestyle and speed jumping. I hadn't jumped rope in three decades, but she taught me that age has nothing to do with one's ability to be fit, healthy and fabulous. She taught me her specialty: "Jumpin' Detox."

Jumping rope is a super fun and exciting exercise that builds aerobic and anaerobic cardiovascular lung capacity. It's a great form of exercise for teenagers and young adult women because it helps build, strengthen, and preserve bones in the body, particularly the bones in the spine and lower legs. Jumping rope is a "plyometric" type of exercise that makes muscles extremely strong and fast, which is needed for sports such as track, tennis, skiing, soccer, and gymnastics. No other exercise will make your legs super strong, super powerful and shapely! Jumping rope burns a bit over 1,000 calories in an hour – it's a fat-blasting incinerator! No other exercise revs up your metabolism the way jumping rope does, plus it improves your hand-eye-foot coordination, balance, agility, timing, and rhythm.

It works both the upper and lower body, giving you one heck of an efficient workout! Everyone can jump rope; young, old, and all fitness levels. You can jump rope anywhere and anytime. Plus, it's cheap. It is fantastic for travel. Every where I go I pack up my "Lucie B" skip rope into my luggage. It is something I can do right in my hotel room. All you need is good pair of cross trainers that absorb shock and a nice springy surface to jump on. Wood, tile, or carpeted surfaces are great. Avoid concrete. Jumping rope can be a bit challenging at first, so work at your own pace, learn and master the basic skills, and build from there.

How Jumping Rope Detoxifies the Body

The human body rids itself of toxins, drugs, and pollution via the lymphatic system. Jumping rope stimulates blood circulation and movement of the lymphatic fluids, detoxifies fatty tissue, and increases lymph flow in the body and flushes waste products and toxins out of the cells. A "detoxified" body is a healthy and stress-free body. Jumping rope helps the blood to circulate efficiently throughout the body, and gives you incredible energy. It also detoxifies the brain by stimulating enzyme activity to increase mental acuity, quickness, and increased reaction time. Skin, muscles, bones and brain...jumping rope works to detoxify and keep a body fit and healthy!

What Jump Rope Should I Get?

You should always begin with a rope you're most comfortable with; beaded ropes are best for beginners. I recommend my beautiful "Lucie B" rope; they are very user-friendly. Each beaded rope is custom made to one's height and weight, so it's not too long or short; the handles have grooves for a good grip, comfort and fluidity of movement. Plus, they are the color of the rainbow, which looks gorgeous when jumping. (See the Grail Boutique at the back of the book to buy your own!)

Fitness Life Plan

- Start by taking little steps.
- Choose a couple of fitness programs that get you excited, and mix it up.
- Seek out and hire the right personal coach or trainer who motivates you.
- Join a fun fitness club, and rearrange your schedule to get there in the morning.
- Remember, keep moving!
- Take a daily walk outdoors, not just for the exercise but for

the connection you regain from the environment each time. It's simply good for the soul!

chapter 6

Know Thyself!

Perception is in the Eye of the Beholder

I must admit I have a great appreciation for being surrounded by beautiful spaces and beautiful things. I am certain that I came into this world with my brain partly wired that way. At least that is my story! And it was my mother's parents who nurtured it whether they knew it or not. It is to them that I owe this obsession which I will not apologize for. When I was a child I was blessed with many summers and holidays spent at my grandparents' home in Germany and at their summer cabin in the area known as Vogelsberg, north of Frankfurt. The cabin was rustic but quaint, with a wood stove to keep warm and a thick feather duvet to get buried in. To me, this was heaven.

My grandfather tended to a wild garden – using his sickle he would clear a maze through overgrown grasses and giant sun-flowers where we got lost in hours of hide-and-seek. In the evenings he would string and light his collection of Chinese paper lanterns and sing lullabies into the night until we couldn't hold our heads up anymore.

I was woken early each morning, sent off with a few coins and a dented old tin container to fetch fresh milk from the local farm, an enormous structure built in the fourteenth century. When I say fresh, I mean I had to stand and watch Frau Muller milk the cow. My grandmother would then boil the milk before we drank it. It was a fairytale scene, a courtyard filled with chickens and roosters, its own brook with a working mill around back. The farm house was three storeys tall, built in traditional half-timber and stucco style framing, with narrow passageways, steep stairwells, and not a straight floor or wall to be found. I also recall the unmistakable odour of cow manure mixed with smells of fresh baked bread. It was, in my mind, the most magical place on earth.

With my grandparents' love for the outdoors we spent our days picking blueberries in the forests and exploring new places. The story of Hansel and Gretel took up space in mind often as we journeyed deep into some of these forests. My grandfather would park his white Volkswagen bug at the bottom of the landscape even if there was a road to the top, which was always our final destination. We climbed by foot up mountains and hillsides to get to the castle, the hidden monastery near my grandparents' home, with secret passageways and hiding places. I remember glimpsing golden chalices and ancient manuscripts, and hearing mythical legends and stories of Lorelei, kings, queens, and Roman invasions. My mind was enraptured by the mystical side of life.

My grandmother was a true lady and one of the kindest, gentlest souls I have ever known. I remember how proud I was of her, always dressed very fashionably and winning "best dressed woman" in the small village outside of Augsburg where they finally retired. They were active and healthy individuals, raising four wonderful daughters. They loved to travel, spending vacation time in places like Baden Baden and other well known mineral spas. They were both diagnosed in their early thirties with heart conditions, but lived into their late eighties. The last time I saw them was in the mid '90s and it was at this time that the first concepts were being developed for Grail Springs. They told me they attributed their health and longevity to their regular trips to the mineral spas.

Though they passed away several years ago now, I have the fondest memories of my life with them. There is no doubt that they and the incredible experiences they bestowed on me, influenced my perception of life, my choices and certainly the outward design and manifestation of what you see today at Grails Springs: a transformation destination for those who seek knowledge and

Know Thyself. A brilliant and exceptional life depends on it.

renewed health. I reflect often on these roots, which have inspired me to keep following my passion, to envision and create beautiful and moving spaces and experiences that add to and inspire other people's lives.

Today I thank Joachim and Herta Wolf – my grandparents – for the creative process in which I thrive; for my healthy curiosity and interest in history, myths and legends, art, and different cultures; for my appreciation for healthy living, all of which I am now so compelled to pass on to others.

Awaken the Observer

How do you perceive life? What state of mind do you create from? Do you perceive and create from a state of joy? Or do you perceive and create from a state of worry? Esther Hicks from the movie The Secret says it so simply. There are only two kinds of feelings in this world: positive and negative. When you observe yourself, does what you are thinking and feeling feel good, or does what your are thinking and feeling feel bad? Paying attention to the state in which you are observing and creating is imperative to the process of self-discovery. Be open to some surprising revelations.

Clearing our heart and mind so that we can begin to create from a place of joy and ease takes a conscious commitment and steadfastness. To detox our mind, our negative thoughts, our habitual negative thinking, all of these things that sabotage our divine state of joy, gratitude, and wellness, we must expect to wake up the observer in ourselves and be willing to look at the deeper meaning of things. The observer is the part of you that can stand apart objectively over you and see what you are thinking, feeling and doing without judgement. You only have to give yourself that command. It will activate. Then focus on the task at hand. Pay attention. The observer is a fundamental component and function of your conscious self.

Once you have discovered it, connect to it, and get it, you won't want to ever leave home without it. Eventually the observer

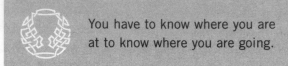

You have to know where you are
at to know where you are going.

just becomes a permanent fixture. I recommend that you invest in a journal and start to keep track of this journey and your "observations." Once you have hit that place on the path where you recognize that it does pay to ask questions and be account-able for what you think, feel, say, and do, something unexpected begins to happen. The mind, the observer, becomes capable of focusing longer and more acutely on those things that you have the desire to know about and understand better. The things that you want to better understand begin to attract themselves towards you so you can have those experiences. What you focus on wanting to know about will appear. Experiences start to show themselves, opportunities start to come fast and furious – this is the Law of Attraction. Through the application of experiencing understanding and then understanding experiences, we gain knowledge, revelations, and actualization. We get to KNOW.

A brilliant and exceptional life, full of originality, depends on you getting to know yourself, your apparatuses like your brain, your mind, your heart, your nervous system, and your chakra system, all of these tools of perception. Inviting your Self, your observer, to start participating consciously will take you on a revelatory journey in self-discovery, the first step to cleansing heart and mind, toxic thinking and feelings, all damaging to your physical body and overall well-being.

Thought is powerful. Imagine a life where there are no obstacles (thoughts) that cause you to feel inadequate, inca-pable, unrecognized, unproductive, untrustworthy, and inferior. Instead, imagine a state of self-certainty that breeds unlimited potential, confidence, independence, creative genius, curiosity, trust, pure joy, and love for life. Imagine a self-trusting, free-flowing mind and heart where decisions and actions come from a place of certainty, spontaneity, ease, and joy, aligning perfectly with your ever evolving vision and goals.

Here is an excellent exercise in self-discovery. Observe the following and write in your journal your findings on these three outward appearances in your life. They can hold a lot of information about you:

- **Association:** What are your relationships like, loving or jealous? What does your family associations look like, dysfunctional or wholesome? Who do you associate with – are they deep or shallow; people with integrity or shady? If you own a business, who have you surrounded yourself with, the best or just adequate? What does your "gang" look like as a whole?

- **Form:** How does your body show up in life – healthy, fit, overweight, anorexic, or suffering ill-health? What does your creation look like – well groomed and cared for, or sloppy and lacking good hygiene? How about your home – is it messy or clean, inviting and warm, or maybe cold and stark? How about your work space – is it chaotic or organized? How about your bank account? What form has that taken? Take a good honest look at all the forms you have created in your life and how they all appear.

- **Realizations:** What have you realized about your life? Are you still guessing about life or are you certain what life is about, particularly your individual life? Do you spend every day conscious and in a state of curiosity, discovery, and revelation? Or do you spend your day allowing your mind to be captivated by entertainment, glued to soap operas, and zoned out? What do you know about life, people, animals, your planet, global warming, and the state of foreign affairs? Have you ever really asked yourself, what does everything I know add up to?

When you have finished the exercise take a good look at the pattern. How hooked up are you to life? How is your connection with all of your surroundings? Clear as a bell, or is there a bit of static most of the time, tuned out, or are you not even interested in getting a dial tone?

How you perceive, think, and feel about life and your environment, is what is manifest on the outside. So maybe you are partially hooked up and plugged in and doing not too bad. Is that good enough for you, or do you think there is room to move further along? Let your inner soul voice become louder. Let your inner soul vision become clearer.

Tips for Journaling

Journaling is an effective tool for contemplative meditation and for accessing your inner thoughts. Your mind can reach into the depths of the Self and allow for free flow of expression. Simply ask yourself a question. Put your pen to the paper and begin writing. It doesn't matter what comes out. Have no judgement about it. Eventually the answer will appear. And, most likely, many more questions.

In a world in which we are so stressed out with the doing of life, going so far as to take our Blackberry to the opera and our laptop on vacation, journaling can be the perfect way to calm life down, take inventory of yourself and your feelings, resolve conflicts, make decisions and bring clarity to mind as well as to record your personal spiritual journey.

- **Right Tools:** Let your writing materials choose you; a beautiful journal and the perfect writing pen.

A good-quality pen that feels comfortable is essential. You want to be able to have an easy, uninterrupted flow.

- **Right Environment:** Find a space that inspires you; a comfortable chair near a window with a view of the sky or trees.

- **Time of Day:** Find a consistent time to write. Don't let a lack of time get in the way. Get up a few minutes early or stay up a few minutes later. Make your journaling practice a priority, a commitment of self-realization and growth.

- **Right Approach:** First, kick out the editor and the critic from your mind. Close your eyes and take a few deep breaths. Become quiet and then allow images and feelings to flow through you. Something will catch your interest. Just put the pen to paper and begin to write about it. Do not spell check and do not worry about style or grammar. Get into that thought and be without hesitation. Be curious, be open, be honest, and be brave.

Meditation
Key to Creation

Meditation is a prerequisite to being an effective creator. It will help you to find the keys to self-discovery, unlock the observer, and to discover the true gifts of vision. Vision is the most powerful ingredient for creation and transformation. Meditation and a focused mind are key. The practice of living life and observing it as one continuous meditation, seeing life wholly from this perspective, is not as difficult as one may think. It is rewarding, and can be integrated into absolutely any lifestyle. Anyone can find their peace of mind, their joy, their enlightenment, their Holy Grail.

Meditation simply means "focused mind." That's it. It is having the capacity to use your mind as you wish, to perceive frequency, rhythms, and thoughts and to transmit frequency, rhythms, and thoughts, creative ideas, concepts, and ideas to the brain.

People have defined meditation as a state of concentration, attention, calm awareness, deep continuous thought, reflection or "being in the zone." You've experienced this many times, just maybe not consciously and not enough of it to achieve the goals and life that you really want, fulfillment both inner and outer.

Those who have dedicated their time and practice to the steady art of meditation say that it can create a permanent heightened sight, can lead to a state of bliss, pure reason, nirvana, and communion with the divine. They gain an ability to tap into truth and certainty.

Most of the guests I get a chance to speak to at Grail Springs tell me that even though they have read about the benefits of meditation, they have avoided the thought of introducing it into their life because in their mind it is something mystical and unattainable. They also can't imagine squeezing one more thing on to their daily "to do" list. I used to think the same way. Luckily for me, I was highly motivated to keep up the practice due to my illness. Admittedly, it took me a very long time, almost ten years, to realize that meditation is not something you "squeeze" in to your schedule like a business call, grocery shopping, or a dentist appointment.

There are three kinds of meditations that can be integrated into your life on a daily basis: silent meditation, invocation meditation, and contemplative or working meditation. In the following pages I will describe some simple methods of approach to get you started. A good exercise for your journal and a good place to start is to first ask some questions of yourself. Why do you think you want to learn to meditate? What would some of your goals be? Some might answer: to reduce stress, learn to relax, improve sleep patterns, heal my body, get re-connected with my body and emotions, my people, my soul, actualize a natural and calm awareness, become more sensitive

[Meditation simply means "focused mind."]

and compassionate, be able to concentrate better, be better at my job, skills, and creative abilities, raise my consciousness, acquire enlightenment. As you can see, there are unlimited benefits to and reasons for learning to meditate. Set goals that are true for you. Then set your mind free from all expectations and old ideas of what you think you should experience. Then be open to receive whatever may come your way. Allow for the surprise because it will surprise you.

I would like to note here to readers and individuals who are well versed in meditation practices that a person can go well beyond what this chapter is proposing. My intent here is to take the mystique out of the subject and guide the novice where they may experience immediate rewards while encouraging ongoing interest and further study. How deep you wish to go "down the rabbit hole" as they say is your choice. I expect to keep discovering new experiences and realization for the rest of my life.

Silent Meditation: A Starting Point

I feel this is a prerequisite for other forms of meditation and I already know some of you are gasping with dread. Relax. Just two minutes a day is all it takes. We're keeping it simple. If you can get really good at silent meditation, it will act as a spring board to catapult you into other forms more easily; invocation and contemplation. Silent meditation is like the spine is to the body. It puts the structure in place that will allow you to eventually break free and do the fun stuff. So let's get started.

1) Find a time that is conducive for quiet and for privacy, perhaps right after dinner each day. Don't do this when you are exhausted. Try to find the time when you are still feeling alert. If you are serious about entering into a deeper inner life, I highly recommend that you create a sacred space for yourself and your family. Make sure you are uninterrupted. For the first little while you will have to control your environment. Tell the spouse, the kids, or housemates not to interrupt you during this time. Unplug the phone if you have to and get comfortable.

2) Sit in a straight back chair. DO NOT lie down. That can come later when you have mastered your meditative life. Place your feet flat on the ground, arms relaxed, palms up. Close your eyes and initiate the observer in you to stand quietly by and watch your thoughts.

3) Take a deep breath. I do not recommend using a mantra when the objective is silence. Instead, on each of the out-breaths, softly and quietly express the sound of "ssshhh." Just as if you are putting a baby to sleep. Repeat over again on each out-breath for approximately two minutes. Eventually you won't have to even express the sound, but you will simply know how to intonate it without any sound at all. What this does is controls the throat chakra. Because the throat chakra (self-talk) is tied to the heart chakra (feelings) and

["Reality is what you are seeking to see and catch and be aware of when you meditate. Meditation is paying un-distractible attention to that which is real."
– Rev. Michael Beckwith, Teacher in the movie *The Secret*]

brow chakra (pictures), once you gain self-control over one, the other two will follow. I have found the throat chakra to be the easiest one to control first.

4) What you will more than likely observe on the in-breath is that a thought and picture will indeed come to mind. It could be something insignificant like a task you forgot to complete that day. When that happens, use your observer to recognize it and dismiss it and continue on. Focus on your throat and your breath and keep this up for the two minutes.

Consider your level of daily commitment. Be realistic and you will succeed. Don't set yourself up for a commitment that is not doable. Even just two minutes a day of quiet meditation is a commendable start and has an immense and powerful effect on your bio-energy field, your chakra system, nervous system, all of your systems, in fact. This process allows for energy input. It is a time to fill-up, to restore your energy tank. It allows for energy input, and energy conservation. When you have mastered silence, you will be able to pose a question, get quiet, be open and listen for the truth that can be revealed.

Utilize available CDs and DVDs on calming techniques, such as breath work, yoga, music, sound therapy, meditation narratives, imaging, or "body scanning." And if you can find one in your area, walk a labyrinth. The goal is that one day you will no longer need to utilize these techniques or tools but will be able to call upon this state of mind at will, even in a crowded room, a football game, driving, etc. There will be no obstacles that will prevent you from having and utilizing this state of calm awareness at will.

Build on this practice and you will find that you will accomplish silence quickly and as you do, you will desire to do more. Then one day you will find yourself sitting in a traffic jam and instead of stressing out, you will go straight in to silent mode and turn your stress around. You'll be able do it in the bank line up or in the boardroom, induce calm just when you need it most. It will become a natural process to want to meditate longer and more often as you go. And your physical body will love you for it. Silence is the greatest healer.

Contemplative Meditation: Open Up to What is Possible

Open up your life to healthy curiosity. Take time to ask questions and be determined to get to the root of the matter. And don't stop there. Ask the next question. What are the possibilities? Talk to yourself like you would counsel a good friend. Sit somewhere quiet and just begin with one single question. See how long you can stick to a subject without getting distracted or bored. A very good method to help you move along which many people find very helpful and therapeutic is journaling every evening before going to sleep. Keep your journal beside your bed and commit to writing five minutes a night to start. You could be pleasantly surprised how writing your thoughts down can concretize what you think you know. You will begin to see a pattern and with this exercise repeated, you will see and understand how to make your dreams reality, you will begin to uncover all kinds of truths about the body, mind, and soul. Hint: thoughtful reflection on the process itself will speed things up.

Invocation Meditation: In Tune with the Universe

To some individuals invocation might be recognized as their prayer life. The output energy of invocation however, would be described as much more potent and present, with a very clear intention and vision. The output of energy contains your own will, co-joining with the universal will. Prayer, which is often in the asking mode, creates room for doubt and uncertainty. Prayer and faith are stepping stones on the path to certain knowing. Invocation demonstrates a person's present knowing and conviction.

This is a very personal endeavour. I have come to revere the power of invocation and use it daily, and mostly spontaneously. On that note however, I have found that there are certain times of day and night, certain times on the moon calendar and seasons when invocation, energy output, can be very potent. It is as though the universe is dialling down to us to hear what we have to say. If you pay attention, pick up, and speak your message very clearly, you will be fully understood and those invocations can start to manifest very quickly. Invocation meditations are your dream boards in action. See your vision clearly, feel it, and feel the rhythm and intention behind it, see it complete, and if you can, see it in motion, three dimensional, feel the physical nature of it, touch it, smell it, hear it, put colour to it (most difficult but will come with practice). Hold it as long as you can and then set it free. I practice this invocation method every single morning before I leave my bed. It is one of several things I do that takes anywhere from 10 to 15 minutes. In that short time I manage to start with some slow deep breathing and silent meditation for just a minute or so, then do some morning stretches (still lying down and most often with a great big smile on my face as I give gratitude for this life), then I prepare my dream board in my mind, make it real, hold it and then let it go, one at a time. Believe me, I always have many things on the drawing board! You can have as many as you want. It is a very fulfilling, efficient and effective way to start any new day and to plan you life. I highly recommend it.

Again, consider that the language of the universe is energy, and behind that moving energy is a frequency, a rhythm. We have found words to define these rhythms of life; humility, for instance which I wrote about earlier. I rarely use words any longer in my invocations. Maybe I will use one word occasionally. Instead, I feel and capture the rhythm of the vision.

Frequencies and rhythms are fluid. They change, and are subject to ebbs and flows. If you don't allow yourself to get stuck in the word, but go beyond and embody the essence of the word, you will begin to tap in to those universal rhythms. Start opening yourself up to what it is that you want. See it clearly. Is it a relationship, is it healing, it is a new career, a dream vacation, a deeper relationship with the universe? The possibilities are endless. As long as your vision is in alignment with the laws of physics, the laws of the universe, you'll be good to go.

Everything in the universe is subject to laws and to their environment at all times. As you become more "in tune" with yourself, your frequency, and your rhythms, you will become more in tune with others and what is affecting them, including the rhythms of the day, people in their life, the seasons, the sun, and the planetary rhythms. There are some very potent moments in time to take advantage of these rhythms for both receiving and invoking. A life of meditation will undoubtedly hook you up to the greatest connection of all, the universe's information highway where you too can get into the flow. I highly recommend a personal subscription to this unlimited network provider!

Vision Manifesting Using Solar Astrology

Solar astrology uses the science of relationships between all living things within the universe. This has proven to be an amazing process in actualizing visions and goals and in my understanding of my personal responsibility and my relationship to the world.

Whether we are conscious of it or not, we are significantly influenced by that which is present around us: environment, weather, people, world events, solar and planetary influences. Being aware of these influences on our psyche can teach us how to connect with our environment to gain positive experiences and outcomes rather than stressful ones. We can move with the ebb and flow of all life, not try to swim upstream against it.

March 21	Spring Equinox
June 21	Summer Solstice
September 21	Autumn Equinox
December 21	Winter Solstice

The practice of solar astrology goes back thousands of years when these solar equinoxes were revered and celebrated. We have been left evidence in stone all over this planet showing us how the Mayans, the Egyptians, the Nordics, and other ancient civilizations worshipped the sun and structured their culture, ceremony and architecture around the cycles of the sun.

The Celts, for instance, celebrated the longest night of the year, December 21st, (referencing the Northern Hemisphere) not because it was the darkest night, but because it marked the rebirth of the sun. Its power, its life-giving energy was returning and that meant the cycle of rebirth was about to begin, a time to prepare for the year to come. It was a time for spiritual growth and realization, symbolically coming out of the darkness and into the light. The two worlds of heaven and earth were recognized and represented as two cords, to be weaven as "One" in the human life experience. The perfect life can be lived by one who successfully awakens and connects to his or her soul reality, the heaven reality, and intertwines this into their earth life, hence creating "heaven on earth." The Celtic Knot is a symbol of this interweaving and for that reason is a part of the Grail Springs logo.

Creating

The full moon in December, preceding the Winter Solstice date of December 21st, is a reminder that we are ending one process and beginning another. On this day thousands of people around the world begin a twofold process of self-reflection and creation. As the sun's energy moves away, we tend to withdraw inwardly, physically, emotionally, and mentally. Mother Nature moves into hibernation mode, a way to store and protect energy reserves through the winter but this winter solstice also gives human beings an opportunity for deep reflection. Some embrace this natural calling, while others find it unnerving. When I look back and remember important people in my life and all of my faithful pets that have come and gone, their illness or condition became worse and/or they passed away during the fall and winter months. It has shown me that the sun's energy plays an integral part of the illness-wellness continuum.

At the winter solstice, I reflect on my accomplishments in the past year, I take an honest accounting as to how well I did and I don't move on until I feel settled and resolved about where I am at with each thing. Following this process, I begin to look at all the new ideas I've collected, open myself up to the creative flow, allowing for input and output of energy, and my vision for the year to come and even beyond. Lists are made and the process begins over again for another year. This is my version of New Year's Resolutions.

Planning

Between Winter Solstice and the Spring Equinox is the planning stage. Symbolically, the fields are prepared, the seeds chosen, help enlisted, protocols prepared, and so on. On March 21st the seeds are planted. This is launch day. This is the day that the plan is implemented. I make sure my "aces are in their places," as a good friend of mine has reminded me on many occasions. Every detail should be understood and everything needs to be where it is supposed to be in order for the launch to be successful, in order for the seeds to take.

Nurturing

The period from launch day to June 21st, the Summer Solstice, is the most laborious of times. This is where the blood, sweat, and tears are shed. And it happens to be a really good time to expend physical energy. Remember that during this time we are shifting closer now to the sun and its energy. We are getting charged by the sun's rays for longer periods each day. All living organisms are receiving more energy. Our water is charged, our food is fresher, and everything is just more alive and abundant.

This is a time to keep a close eye on the plan. Nurture the vision, water it, feed it, and fertilize it. We wait for those seeds to pop and show the first signs that we might be on to something. And when the first harvest finally arrives by June 21st, it should bring forth the recognition that we have either done a good job and can expect further growth or the lack of it will tell us that we either didn't think something through or maybe our heart just wasn't in it completely. If we did well, we get to enjoy the fruits of our labour.

Now we are entering mid-summer and the sun is beginning to withdraw. It is hot, so we tend to relax just a little, celebrate a little, go on summer vacations, and spend some of our earnings or profits while we await the second harvest.

Accounting

By the third quarter, September 21st, just like the Celts, I am gathering and storing all the fruits of my labour. I'm planning ahead how to utilize it best, how to share and where to spread it around, and begin to already look at what was really successful and what could be done differently. New ideas most certainly have been born. I expect it. I keep records of all new inspirations, because by the full moon in December I know I am starting the process all over again.

Through this conscious process it never ceases to amaze me as to what I have been able to actualize, and I am convinced that solar astrology speeds up manifestation and attracts opportunities. Whether we are aware of it or not, the human psyche is influenced by this powerful source called the sun.

You don't need to wait until the end of the year to get started. You can enter into the process today and just start to pay attention to the influence of your environment on yourself, your children, your partners, and your colleagues.

Here are some guidelines to follow throughout the year

STEP 1: Purchase a "Manifesting Journal" and make sure this journal is only used for the purposes of making your dreams and goals realities. Make it small enough that you can travel around with it, in your purse, car or briefcase. A lap top will work as well.

STEP 2: Full moon in December – take an accounting, "did I accomplish what I set out to do this year? And how well did I do it?" There is usually one major accomplishment that stands out plus many smaller ones. What did you learn that was a complete surprise? What do you have to be grateful for? If you ask the right questions, the answers can be pearls of wisdom. If you don't ask the right question, you can be left in the dark. Gratitude and realization are both keys to your desired future.

STEP 3: Look towards the coming year. What's your passion? Get clear about what you want. This usually has already been brewing and is at the forefront of your mind. If you are focused, you will see the possibilities. When it feels right, THAT is the inspired thought and that is the one that should be acted upon. HINT: The answers or response you get, will always match your level of passion!

STEP 4: Make New Year's Eve a special night for YOU. At some point go sit alone somewhere and light some candles, get quiet and collect your thoughts. Make your commitment to YOU. Say it out loud. Read your list of things that you desire to accomplish. For me, it includes one BIG thing, and many smaller things. Say it all, get it all out. And when you are done, be done. Then go have a great time with your friends and family. Celebrate the passing of the old, and the welcoming of the new!

STEP 5: The first day of the year, be ready to align yourself with your new goals and visions. What's the plan? What, who, where, and when all have to be answered. You have to be ready for launch day. Aces in their places!

STEP 6: March 21st – launch your plan. Work at it and keep your eyes on the outcome. Keep the vision all the while you are doing what needs to be done to make it happen.

STEP 7: June 21st – take a good look as to what is growing. Have you a healthy first harvest? What more can you do? But don't forget to take time to rest, play, and enjoy the fruits of your labour.

STEP 8: Sept 21st – assess, preserve, disperse, reflect, account.

STEP 9: During the full moon in December you start it all over again, beginning with a final accounting and opening yourself up to new creations.

STEP 10: Take a few minutes at the beginning of each day to review how you are doing. It will bring forth new ideas to act upon and many surprises that you can't even imagine were possible. Through this wonderful process you will begin to feel a stronger connection with your surroundings. You'll begin to figure out how things work, and you will soon learn how to always be in the flow of life where your creative energy can be optimized.

As you begin to manifest the life you want, consider your well-being, your family's well-being, and the well-being of your planet. Everyone and everything should be included in your vision. If you want to have a brilliant, joyful, and abundant life, make sure your health and the health of your planet is considered in the picture. We hope these ideas from Grail Springs will help you achieve your perfect life, both physically and soulfully.

Here is a list of some ideas to start with. I call these "my baskets." And I try to pay as much attention to one as I do to the others. You will find that if you put too much energy into one basket, another will pay. Find balance, and keep it balanced.

Exercise: The New Beginning
What do you wish to begin to manifest now in your life to ensure wholeness and happiness forever?

Consider:

Education	Health
Relationships	Professional
Finances	Play
Soul	Hobby
Your Community	Planet
Philanthropy	Other

The Labyrinth
Sacred Tool for Meditation

The labyrinth was created in ancient times and it represents humankind's search for the core of divinity. The labyrinth pattern is an archetypal form found all over the world. It dates back at least 3,500 years. No one knows who created the original labyrinth form as it appears in many civilizations such as India, Egypt, Crete, Scandinavia, Italy, and many others. We do know that embedded within each design is a flow in pattern that when

[
"Unlike a maze whose intent it is to get us lost, the labyrinth is designed to get us found."
– Unknown
]

properly engaged, can induce calm awareness, healing, as well as take us to our deepest inner self where we can hear our own wisdom and our soul's wisdom attempting to reach us.

The circular shape symbolizes the universe, wholeness and unity. We, the observer, can take ourselves into the depths of this world. Whether walked on or traced in sand, the labyrinth pattern is a powerful tool for reflection, invocation, meditation, healing, bringing calm and a deeper knowledge of the true Self.

Unlike a maze, a labyrinth is made up of one singular linear path that begins from the outer edge, directing the participant into a heart centre, and then returns them back to the outer edge by following the same route they took to get in. It is a three part process. The outside represents our earthly life, and the centre represents our heavenly life, our soul, and the totality representing the entire universe.

Through the act of trusting the path, of giving up conscious control of how things should go and being receptive to our inner state, we can be opened up to a whole new world of insight, inspiration, and creation. Through following the beautiful flow of these sacred patterns, labyrinths help us to ground ourselves. Some people experience a state of timelessness and find this type of surrender particularly relaxing and renewing.

Grail Springs Sacred Labyrinth: The Knight's Connection
In medieval times, the labyrinth became the symbol of the spiritual pilgrimage to the Holy City of Jerusalem, not exclusive to any one religious order but to all of those whose centres resided

there. Jerusalem is considered the heart of the labyrinth. This quest, or focused walk to the centre of the City of Jerusalem was for serious spiritual reflection and contemplation. Answers, revelation, and inspired thought were expected to come once the journeyers had reached inside their temple located in the Holy City of God. The Knights Templar were protectors of these routes, allowing safe passage for anyone who wished to make the trek.

After arriving at their destination and after several weeks of rest, recuperation, and preparation, it was time to make the trek back home, also an intent-filled journey of contemplation to discover how they would now implement their discoveries or realizations into their lives, their families, their villages, and their people. In other words, what was their plan? This is where human will is expected to step in, and this of course is what separates those who have great inspirations, from those who act on their great inspirations.

When the Knights Templar left their headquarters in Jerusalem in 1187 it became more and more dangerous for individuals to travel and make the spiritual quest to the city. It was the Knights Templar and their fellow questers the Freemasons who adopted the four quadrant, eleven circuit labyrinth as the most sacred shape in the universe. They began to finance and build sacred architecture including labyrinths all over the European continent, so that individuals could symbolically make their spiritual journey and connection with the Holy City of God. They built Chartres Cathedral in France in 1201 as a repository for ancient wisdom. Chartres includes the most famous labyrinth in the world, and the one most replicated, including at Grail Springs.

An interesting fact about the history of labyrinths is that early on they were favoured by the Roman Catholic Church and existed within many of the Gothic Cathedrals that were built between the twelfth and thirteenth centuries. However, by the seventeenth century, the Roman Catholic Clergy decided for whatever reason that the labyrinths were to be destroyed and that is exactly what took place. All but one was destroyed, Chartres in France. The clergy were afraid to destroy this one in particular and so left it untouched but they did cover it with chairs so no one could walk it. Some have speculated that they began to recognize that the labyrinth was allowing the individual direct access to the main source, the big guy in the sky, and the god within us all. The threat of this became too real to the hierarchal organization of the church. It is because of this one small act, to leave the Chartres labyrinth intact, that we are lucky enough now to see a renaissance revival of this sacred device.

Interpretations of the circuits surrounding the centre include that they represent the solar system with the centre representing the sun, each circuit a representation of the power or attributes of the surrounding planets. Another is that the labyrinth represents the human body, in particular the chakra system as taught through the different yoga schools. There are many different representations of labyrinths around the world.

Community of Labyrinth Seekers Around the World

In our present day we are rediscovering the labyrinth as the spiritual tool that it is. Many communities are coming together to construct labyrinths in their city parks. Churches are installing them for prayer and contemplation and for finding one's way through difficult times; spiritual centres are creating them for those on retreat, and hospitals and hospices are building labyrinths for patients, encouraging that they walk the labyrinth before surgery or while recovering from illness.

Perhaps you can find a labyrinth somewhere within your community. If you do an online search, you will be amazed at the large community of labyrinth walkers, researchers, and builders. I encourage you to take a journey on one. Go as often as you are moved to go. Allow your natural curiosity to come forth. The labyrinth is a tool for meditation. We know meditation is simply the art of "focusing your mind's attention with a calm awareness." Your Intention is a key to your success.

The labyrinth can be approached using three methods of meditation. You may simply want to utilize it for a silent meditation – to think nothing at all. Just to experience peace of mind, freedom from the inner voice of chatter. This is a great way to start if it is your first time and it is also great for balancing and stimulating healing energy. Take some deep breaths and just walk gently and slowly. You may want to use it for visualizing a healing for someone you know, even yourself. Many people say that this experience provides the most powerful feeling of being focused and connected.

You may wish to use it for a working meditation or contemplative meditation, for creative uses, for building ideas, problem solving, for getting answers about decisions you are facing, or for figuring out life's unending mysteries. The experience and outcome is very surprising to most.

Walking the Sacred Labyrinth

As you sit outside the circle, focus your thoughts on what you want to accomplish. Ask yourself what it is that you would most like to know, most like to have assistance with. Try not to have any preconceived ideas. Prepare yourself. Calm yourself. Empty your mind of chatter, your heart of any anxiety. Start with a few deep breaths, relax and enjoy the simplicity of the experience.

When you feel ready, begin your walk. Taking slow, small and steady steps is a good start, but there are no rules. You may at times just feel like stopping. You may feel like sitting down in the middle of your walk to contemplate something you just discovered or to regroup. You may also feel like leaving and going to sit down outside of the circle again. You may feel like starting over. Again, there are no rules. What you will find is that long after you are done, you will continue to realize even more about the actual experience and all of its subtleties.

If you are doing an invocation meditation, relax and find your silence first, bring up your intention, and begin to express your desire. Keep your intent in the forefront of your mind and heart. That is where you want to persist in your focus. The universe responds to energy produced by your rhythm, and it communicates with energy so be prepared to respond to the rhythm. Positive energy attracts positive energy. Negative energy attracts negative energy. The spoken word carries in it your intentions and intention translates into energy – the universal language. So remember, your intent is more important than your actual words.

Don't worry if you feel awkward or stumble at first, or you don't feel like it is flowing well and you are not poetic enough. Modesty is perfectly acceptable. Hint - Humility in your expression is a key to "getting connected." There is no judgment here.

The more you open up your mind and embrace a daily practice of meditation, whether you do yoga, use tools such as journaling, or are able walk a labyrinth, the more you do, the more confidence you will gain, and eventually you will begin to get into a permanent rhythm. You will feel "connected" with everything around you and that is a very satisfying place to be. Being more connected to your Self, your body, universal intelligence, life, Mother Nature, humanity, your family, and friends can be the reward. And greater sense of "meaningfulness" will overwhelm you every single day for the rest of your life.

Creating Sacred Spaces

In November 2004 I was on retreat in California about two hours south of Los Angeles. The property sat in a valley surrounded by rolling rills, vineyards, herbs and vegetable gardens. One morning I received a call from home. It was not good news. Removing myself from the workshops for the day I decided to go for a long walk to clear my mind. The garden path which led up the hillside seemed like a good place to start, to get some solitude and to think about how I was going to fix things. As I approached the crest of the hill, a beautiful labyrinth appeared in front of me. Its wide rings looked like a perfect beaded neck-lace of pearls, smooth river rocks gently embedded in the soft sand. This was only the second labyrinth I had come across in my lifetime, the first having been in Paris. Paris sparked my curiosity about labyrinths, but it was this labyrinth in California that was about to deliver to me an invaluable golden key, a key that would unlock a most powerful and profound revelation I soon came to understand that this insight was based on univer-sal principles and laws held by many seers and sages of the past and present, including the labyrinths' original devoted guardians, financiers and builders, the Knights Templar, the Freemasons and the Alchemists.

I confess, I have been bonded to the sacred labyrinth ever since that day. I revere it as a living thing, and have a great sense of affinity and stewardship for its gifts, its magic and continued existence. In fact, as I write this new chapter I am envisioning that Grail Springs has convinced the planners for our town revi-talization project to build a sacred labyrinth out of the local min-erals it is so famous for, as the anchor for the new public spaces, gardens and walkways in Bancroft. The labyrinth at Grail Springs, based on the labyrinth at Chartres in France, has been well walked by many a guest (and myself) for the past ten years, and is a great source of inspiration and peaceful meditation.

Researching the sources and the history of the sacred labyrinth brought many curious thoughts about sacred design, sacred num-bers, sacred alchemy and sacred geometry to mind. These were terms I was somewhat familiar with from art history classes many years ago. In high school I was assigned a paper on the Italian Architect Andrea Palladio, one of the most influential architects of the 15th Century. Starting out as a young stone mason, he became knowledgeable in sacred geometry, the harmonic proportions of music and the Golden Ratio, a mathematical formula which is considered to produce the most aesthetically pleasing form to the human eye and ear.

All of his designs were based on the sacred, all boasting balance and harmony above all and he grew to become a much sought after architect by the rich and famous patrons of Italy. Most of the masters of the Renaissance era came to know, embrace, paint, create music and build magnificent architecture based on these very sacred formulas, from Palladio, to DaVinci, to Chopin. There may be a formula for creating balance and harmony, but as we all know, it still takes skill, will and thoughtful practice to make it happen.

The process of building the labyrinth at Grail Springs prompted me to ponder further; what else makes a space sacred? And who makes it so? I walked our new labyrinth for months and months, continuing to ponder this question over and over, letting it incubate.

In my travels, I have been fortunate enough to have touched or been in the presence of sacred relics and have visited sacred places around the world, from cathedrals, Pharaoh's tombs and battlefields, to the Holy Sepulchre in Jerusalem. As I continued to meditate, I began to capture the following understanding; a sacred or holy place is any 'space' where heart and mind is willing to embody a 'state of reverence'.

The term 'reverence' means to have a sense of honour, respect and awe all at the same time for something greater than you. This state urges or produces an action of peace, harmlessness and benevolence. It can induce a higher purpose or calling, and ultimately can fire up a direct connection with the divine. As part of this, a very unusual feeling can well up inside, a strong feeling to serve and protect. It can take you by surprise. And this followed by a spontaneous urge and conviction to take a vow. This act, even if taken internally, quietly and with no seeming witnesses, acts as a seal. That is, it now becomes 'sacred', a sacred oath. You've left your stamp or your footprint, forever. It carries with it the power of manifestation, the power of communion with the divine, your will and divine will working together. I do believe that it is this very powerful act which leaves your imprint as residual energy for others to sense and feel after you yourself have long gone.

To build on this idea I'd like to refer back to March 2006 when I attended a retreat on the high history of the Grail from the Templar perspective. It was fascinating. What was brought to my attention was the observance of ceremony and sacred relics, and their relevance to spiritual inspiration, vision, revelations and enlightenment including the relics or ceremonies' hidden powers to induce spontaneous healing. This explained some unanswered questions regarding some of the most unusual experiences I have had while traveling and visiting sacred places. The Templars placed great importance on the idea of protecting sacred relics and spaces. They strongly believed that if you meditated while in the presence of these places or things, you could absorb their gifts, impressions and even their realizations.

Whether a person is a 'believer' or a 'non-believer', we hear of individuals often feeling spiritually moved when encountering a historical relic or entering a holy place. Those who are intuitive would say that that they can sense the previous stewards of the space or of the relic itself. There are many religious festivals around the world that have named an annual date to revere and celebrate a sacred place, a sacred relic, or a person such as a saint. There is usually a ceremony followed by great festivity.

Celebration can be quite powerful in changing group consciousness. The world recently witnessed this with the January 20th, 2009 inaugural ceremony and celebration of the first African-American President of the United States, Barrack Obama. Coincidentally the day before this historical inauguration was Martin Luther King Day, a national day of celebration.. With these two significant days landing back to back, hundreds of millions of people around the world were swept up in this high energy which inspired unity, service and self-responsibility, creating potential for great change in the world.

"Ceremony engages the individual to focus all of their attention for that moment towards the object, to give honour to that place or person, with the intent to embody the very attribute or message they represent."

Ceremony is considered a sacred act in every culture, religion and tradition. It is designed to invoke an experience in realization that will benefit the participant. Ceremony engages the individual to focus all of their attention for that moment towards the object, to give honour to that place or person, with the intent to embody the very attribute or message they represent, *and become like it.* This is also an act of meditation that usually involves all three types of actions; silence, contemplation and invocation.

The natural question that followed next for me was; why couldn't I create a sacred space, in my home, in the garden, in the labyrinth or even inside Grail Springs itself? For me, the ultimate quest as a designer is to create divine design. In fact, for me the question keeps getting bigger and bigger and soon becomes quite altruistic: why couldn't our entire planet be renovated into one big sacred space; an extreme makeover of the ultimate kind! Imagine that, everyone waking up every morning and having reverence for something greater than themselves. Hmmm… perhaps by the afternoon it would be a different world?

I've used several spaces in my home over the years to practice meditation, yoga and the Grail Morning Mantra, but finally I settled on creating a permanent and sacred space in my bedroom. I first started to put to paper the vision for my home during the early stages of pregnancy with my son Michael, sitting for months on end at my drafting table imagining every single nook and cranny, making certain that every corner of our home was going to be inviting, nurturing and inspiring.

One of the most important design rules that I learned in college was: 'Form follows function.'

When designing any space I would place myself inside the imaginary room. I would imagine the function that I could see myself or a family member performing in that room, and I would watch as the form would start to appear. I would attempt to bring the exact size of the room to scale inside my mind's eye: the colours, the fabrics, textures and furnishings. I would picture what the room would look like flooded in evening and morning light, both natural and incandescent. It had to function as well as take beautiful form. As long as I stuck to that rule, it usually worked out. There were of course budget restrictions, but I was pretty good at balancing and compromising.

At the time I didn't recognize this process as meditation itself. But that is exactly what it was. I used this process to design and build both Grail Springs and my home. Today, sixteen years later, I still love and adore my home and all the spaces at Grail Springs. Every time I enter the Great Hall, even all these years later, I am in awe. And when I return home from a business trip, I feel true joy stepping across its threshold. My son and I often give a big shout out "we love our home!". And nothing pleases me more than to see my son feeling the same way. As parents I think most of us hope to create a loving, safe and inspiring environment for our children to grow in. Their home should be a sacred space.

This leads me to my greater vision, which is that architects, designers and new home developers in the near future will incorporate a special room in every residence specifically designated for meditation, a space which becomes the central most important feature in the family home. These spaces will purposefully be designed for inner reflection, calm, healing, rejuvenation, meditation and creativity, for the well-being of the whole family. And not just in homes, but in public areas such as schools, seniors' homes, government buildings, offices, parks, and most importantly hospitals, which I hope one day we can refer to as wellness centres instead.

The movement towards this vision is already starting, with individuals building green, eco-friendly homes, incorporating spa-inspired bathrooms, meditation gardens and even small yoga studios into their new home designs. Many corporate companies now enlist the assistance of a certified Feng Shui practitioner to analyze their office space and make recommendations on how to optimize the function of their space for the wellbeing of their staff and clients. Productivity and revenue can increase significantly as a result.

I have had both my business and my home Feng Shui certified and I can tell you there was a notable shift for the better once I made the recommended changes. Feng Shui is an ancient Chinese method that is considered a precise science. Experts use specific formulas to recognize the flow of energy, both positive and negative forces – yin and yang-- as they move and relate to and through the environment, inclusive of both the exterior and the interior of the space. It's a way of ensuring that the energy is balanced, allowing it to move freely in and out of that space. This has a significant effect on the human psyche and ultimately on our health. Build a labyrinth in your back yard, at the cottage, or create a space indoors. Either way, just find one place to create your sacred space indoors and out.

Tune in and use your own intuition to create these spaces. The purpose here is to create a space that inspires you towards the journey of self-realization and well-being. Children are drawn to these kinds of spaces like magnets. Your whole family will benefit from this creation.

Here are some tips for creating your own sacred space:

Transform one room to start: perhaps there is a spare bedroom in your house that you are no longer using. How about transforming that wasted formal dining room that no one has used since the 1960's except to host the annual Thanksgiving dinner? If there is no extra space then perhaps choose a happy corner in a room that could potentially lend itself; perhaps your bedroom or a study. I say happy corner because again, you want to choose an area that feels pleasant, not confined. And may I offer this additional advice — do NOT choose your home office where the computer is! This mediataion/relaxation room should be free from computers, televisions, electronic games and digital clocks. It must be a time-free zone. The only exception will be a cd player for your relaxation music.

Start fresh: Strip the room. Wipe the slate clean. Remove all of its contents and give it a good cleansing. And don't put anything back just yet. Clear the energy in the space by burning a sage stick or some incense.

Pick a colour(s) that move your soul: Choose a colour that doesn't irritate you but rather makes you go 'aahhhhhh'. If you are having difficulty choosing, look through some magazines and every time you see a photo with a colour that makes you feel good and calm, tear it out. Eventually you will start to see a pattern of what you like. Pay attention to the depth of the colour, tones and hues. You want to feel at peace every time you step into the space. Here are some general positive attributes of colour in regards to space but ultimately you need to use your intuition when it comes to choice:

- White   Newness, purity, innocence
- Yellow   Optimism, stimulation, cleanliness
- Orange   Joy, communication, concentration
- Red   Prosperity, warmth, strength
- Purple   Spiritual, passion, motivation
- Pink   Purity, warmth, joy
- Blue   Peace, mystery, contemplation
- Green   Harmony, healing, freedom

Lighting: Every professor, architect and designer that ever taught me in school all agreed on one thing, lighting was the most important element in the design of a space. You could change the entire feel of a space by simply adjusting the light. Natural light is best. Filters such as muslin or stained glass on the windows can make for nice diffusers and add to the atmosphere. And candlelight and firelight always warms the soul.

Soft, minimal furnishings and textures: Keep this room airy, soft and beautiful. A few meditation pillows on the floor and a yoga mat to inspire some movement are a good start. Be conscious of the fabrics and texture you are bringing in to the room. Make sure everything you bring in feels good and make you say 'aaahhhh'. You want your fabric choices to be yummy to the touch too.

Surround yourself with beautiful things that have meaning to you and inspire you: Build a personal altar if you are so moved. The purpose of an altar is to bring focus. For instance, you can build an altar for healing, for motivation, for creativity or for a positive outcome to something. I have a few special gifts given to me from close friends such as a chime, a statue, and a scarf which drapes over my altar, and special trinkets that come from my travels including rocks from other sacred spaces. Yes I confess. I have been known to remove rocks, rubble and sand for my collection from sacred places, but with great respect and reverence! These small objects stir beautiful memories, inspirations and visions of being right there again. I checked with my conscience and it was more than okay!

Visit daily: Start your day and end your day with a visit to your sacred space. Even just for five minutes. Light a candle, burn some incense, play the Grail Mantra, do some yoga, meditate and create a ceremony of your own. Fill your cup and pass it on to your family and friends. For the truth is, we are all sacred.

chapter 7
Conclusion
The Grail Life Guide

As I write the final chapter for this book, I am still feeling charged by memories of the final days of my stay in the Orkney Islands of Scotland. I had awoken early on the last day to clear blue skies and several wild rabbits outside the window. The bed and breakfast we were staying at peered over the sloping fields towards Scapa Flow, a natural harbour used by the Nordics, a thirteenth century Viking king, the Knights Templar, and the British fleets of both world wars. It wasn't hard to imagine these historic scenes, a vivid reminder of the circle of life continuum. Everything must change.

I said my goodbyes to this beautifully haunting place rich in Nordic history including family heritage, this place that had captured my heart and soul for reasons I didn't really understand until just a few days previous. After a two hour ferry crossing back to the mainland, my son and I scrambled down the breathtaking coastal highway for a chance meeting with the International Grand Prior of the Order of The Gnostic Templars, Ian Sinclair, and Malcolm Sinclair, Earl of Caithness and Chief of the Clan Sinclair. Our destination was Noss Head, three miles outside of the town of Wick. We were told to look for the lighthouse. It really does pay to know where you are at in order to know where you are going. All I can say is thank goodness for "Tom Tom" our rented and reliable GPS tracking device!

Finally, the white lighthouse standing alone appeared out of the sandy dunes. Ian Sinclair resides there. It also houses the Clan Sinclair Study Centre and Library. The Sinclair family has a significant connection to the Orkney Islands, the history of Rosslyn Chapel, and the Grail as it relates to the Knights Templar. The library is a treasure trove of rare books, records, prints, initiatory swords, and Templar talismans. As Ian, a tall handsome Highlander with a melodic Scottish brogue, shared stories of Rosslyn and the Holy Grail, he easily captured the imagination of my ten-year-old son Michael, and I knew we were here for him. As I stood with great satisfaction witnessing this wonderful exchange between young and old, I was reminded of my life's ongoing and compelling quest for discovery that was first stirred by my grandfather. It was a very satisfying moment. Admittedly, I believe the face of Sean Connery might have popped into mind for one brief moment!

Life is a journey. My journey is not unlike yours or anyone else's. There is a happy ending to this story. I am forever grateful that my mother, my father, my brother, and I were able to heal ourselves from cancer, alcoholism, depression, anxiety, divorce and from disconnection from ourselves. Not only did my father fully recover, at seventy years of age, he is now our right-hand man at Grail Springs. He is head of maintenance – you'll find him tossing hay to the horses every single morning without fail – and is affectionately thought of by both guests and staff. Though diagnosed with diabetes a few years ago, he impresses me with his dutiful care for his own health, never missing his regular check ups and continually getting a clean bill of health.

Every day and every moment we are on that path of opportunity for discovery and for restoration. We arrive, we live, we get lost, we resist, and we get sick. Somewhere along the line we may stop resisting, we may find an open window, and we may start to make a conscious change. Restoration and transformation is possible for everyone. The journey in self-discovery is a rite of passage, a coming-of-age into our own awakening consciousness and realization of the co-creatorship we can command for our life; in health and well-being. And that is the perfection of life. Triumph over tribulation is the quest and it is the promise of the Grail. I sought, I found, and I drank from the cups; now I am obliged to pass it onto you. My hope is that in some way, this book has provided you with some new thoughts and ideas that you may embrace into your life and your family's life and that through some of these practices you heal, you thrive, and you live the "perfect and brilliant life."

Grail Life Guide

This quick-glance guide has been provided for you on "The 7 Elements of the Grail Life." Many of these lessons I have gathered over the years, shared by many great teachers, coaches, and inspirational speakers and who I have to thank eternally for passing their cup unto me:

Assess

I know where I am at so I know where I am going.

- be self-responsible for your own health and well-being
- have the courage to be honest and accountable to yourself and others
- enlist the support of a Naturopath to guide you on your holistic journey
- know what point you are at on the illness-wellness continuum
- take the Grail Springs online wellness test and track your progress
- raise your standard after every achievement

Cleanse

I wipe the slate clean constantly.

- adopt a seasonal detox regimen
- be keenly aware of the toxicity levels of food, environment, emotions and how you think
- forgive everybody

Nourish
I nourish body, mind,
and spirit.

- adopt the acid/alkaline pH balance approach to your diet
- listen to your body and give it what it needs to carry you through a long and brilliant life

Move
I am fit, I am strong,
and I keep my energetic
system charged.

- enlist a personal fitness coach who inspires you
- feel strong, be strong
- play!

Breathe
I breathe life deeply.

- create an oxygen-friendly environment in home, car, and work space
- breathe deeply, breathe clean
- take in the fresh outdoors often

Think
My soul is my vehicle
for transformation and
manifestation. My mind
is the tool that wields it.

- allow the presence of gratitude in at all times
- nurture you mind with new ideas regardless of where they come from
- embrace solitude
- be both a student and a teacher for life
- meditate
- envision with clean, healthy, rich, inspired thoughts, and you will manifest a clean, healthy, rich, and inspired life
- wield and transform energy for the purpose of raising consciousness

Support
I back myself up
completely.

- care deeply about your life
- be masterful at everything you do
- turn your "should do" into "I have done it"
- be your passion and express your conviction
- turn your home and work place into a healthy and sacred place
- invite your soul to be present at all times
- connect with the universal life-force
- honour and respect all life
- visit somewhere new in the world every year to expand your view of the world
- be well so the planet can be well
- and never stop asking yourself "what are the possibilities?"

Acknowledgements

I would like to acknowledge the following individuals with whom I have had the privilege of sharing this incredible journey: my brother Andrew, my mother Barbara, and my father William. Thank you for granting me creative licence to speak openly about our family struggles so that others might overcome theirs.

To my teachers, mentors, and friends all over the world who cheer me on and hold the light themselves, thank you. You share in the vision that this world can indeed flourish in harmony and live in peace forever.

I thank the "Girls Club": Anita, Lynne, Dorrie, and Diana, who taught me the importance of nurturing your friendships and what a good old-fashioned belly laugh can do for your well-being.

Thanks to John Braunisch for your infectious enthusiasm towards fitness. You've uncovered and shown me so many layers that I didn't know existed. To our fabulous contributing kitchen crew at Grail Springs who designed the recipes for *Grail Springs Holistic Detox*: Melissa and Keith Friesen, Nancy Howard, and Canadian Olympic gold medalist chefs Rebecca Hutchings and Tommy Archibald. A special acknowledgement to Patty James Organic Cooking School in California who provided much inspiration and many incredibly yummy and healthy recipes. Outstanding job, all of you!

I thank Lauretta Hayes for reminding me once in a while to nurture what already is, when I'd rather be off creating what could be. To Liz Baughman, a sister-in-arms, who also provided many of the juicing recipes for this book, who brings unconditional love and endless healing energy to people and planet. I thank my friend Dr. Elson Haas for giving clarity to this book and for showing us what the future of medicine could look like.

Thank you Kim McArthur, my publisher and editor, for entering the door of Grail Springs exactly one year ago. You saw the vision, you invested in it, and you've helped to change the future for the better. You are an extraordinary example of what a woman looks like who embodies both grace and strength. I thank you for taking this book to a whole other level. I am grateful to the staff at McArthur & Company Publishing for backing this book with their creative skills and supportive enthusiasm.

And to the incredible team here at Grail Springs who are heroes everyday, including my personal assistant Melissa MacDonald for making order out of my sometimes whirlwind life. To all of those in the past who gave of their labour and love, often going beyond the call of duty and demonstrating the true spirit of service, the true spirit of the Grail. To our guests and clients at Grail Springs who support the vision by trusting us everyday

Finally, to my son, Michael Marentette, for also teaching me something (which I am still trying to figure out). You keep the mystery alive in our house and I love you for it. I am enjoying every moment of discovering who you are.

Index

Recipe Index

Grail Springs Testimonials

Einstein said, "To do the best we can is our sacred human responsibility." That is precisely why I frequent Grail Springs. From the moment one enters it is obvious a high intelligence has orchestrated a life changing experience, one that surpasses other world class spas. Renewal occurs in ways one would never imagine. I strongly suspect the Grail is in the charge of the angels, and Madeleine Marentette their maestro.

— Gloria Evangelista, award-winning author

I'm still glowing from our weekend at Grails Springs! I'm looking at last weekend as a new beginning, with a renewed sense of purpose and focus on wellness. Ann and I totally love Grail Springs, and the experience exceeded our expectations in every way. Best of luck with your book — I can't wait to read it!

— M. Meredith

I was here two years ago and knew I would return often. Grail is a very special experience. Each time I have had a transformation and have been able to incorporate the lessons and reflections into my life. Great additions and changes- love the evening lectures and Madeleine's involvement. Excellent touch! The experience gets better and better. Thank you all.

— B. Diclemente

I feel like I grew emotionally, mentally, spiritually, and physically to a place I wanted to be for a long time and was unable to reach on my own. With the help of all the people who were here I have now reached a place of inner peace and have tools to continue fine tuning. Thank you so much.   — Jesse

When I came to Grail Springs my expectations were some yoga, some healthy eating, and some treatments that are all new to me. What I got from Grail Springs was way beyond my expectations. Both physical and mental. I am a changed man, much gratitude to you all. — R. Bird

This was a 10 day transformation I will never forget — physical and emotional! Thank you all! — Y. Krotky

Once again my stay gladdened my heart — I am well on my way to feeling fit and strong! Thank you! — N. Carswell

This slice of heaven (Grail Springs) is how the world should look and be — accessible to everyone. — N. Leytes

Grail Spring is the perfect place for a respite to tune into your inner self. If you partake in the Grail you will gain a sense of balance and wellness in your life mentally, physically, and emotionally. I still smile when I think of the Grail!

— M. Kowalewski

Total life changing experience for me. I can't thank everyone enough for all the love, support, and friendships developed.

— A. Van deRoest

It was an awakening to self love and a healthy living for me. I have learned the importance of cleansing my internal body through juicing, exercise, colonics, along with numerous exceptional treatments. The entire staff is so gracious and attended to my every need. Certified therapists embrace all guests with gentleness and a sincere caring attitude. My stay at Grail Springs felt like being in a beautiful soft cocoon; nurtured and groomed for the final transformation. — K. Nutter

Through the lifestyle and diet changes I made as a result of my visit to Grail Springs I have been able to control my Lupus, an auto-immune disease. Since that first visit I have not taken any medication nor had symptoms. I believe this is a result of following the alkaline balanced diet and regular detoxifying treatments that I learned at Grail Springs. Thank you, thank you.

– J. Bailey

The Grail Boutique

Everything mentioned in *Grail Springs Holistic Detox* – from books to spa products to Lucie B's jump ropes – are available at the Grail Springs Boutique and can be ordered through our online store: www.grailsprings.com.